The Adventures of
Swamp Woman

Menopause: Essays on the Edge

The Adventures of Swamp Woman

Menopause: Essays on the Edge

By

Ferida Wolff

authorHOUSE™

1663 LIBERTY DRIVE, SUITE 200
BLOOMINGTON, INDIANA 47403
(800) 839-8640
WWW.AUTHORHOUSE.COM

First published by AuthorHouse 10/25/04

ISBN: 1-4208-0237-2 (e)

Library of Congress Control Number: 2004097501

Printed in the United States of America
Bloomington, Indiana

This book is printed on acid-free paper.

For Harriet May Savitz
who courageously blazes new paths at every age
and generously shares her trials, knowledge, and
caring,
with my love
And for my menopausal sisters
also with love

Table of Contents

Foreword

There are a lot of edgy, transitional women out there. I am one of them. With nearly thirty-two million of us today and an estimated forty-five million by the year 2020 on the frontlines of menopause battling hot flashes, night sweats, heart palpitations, mood swings, and sleepless nights, there is a need for acknowledgement, understanding, and most of all honesty about a major change in women's lives.

Life sneaks up on us when we aren't looking. As children we feel we're pushing against a headwind and can't wait to grow up, as elders we're reaching back for our youth. In between we are a large population of very confused people. Twenty-somethings are still playing around with priorities. Thirty-year-olds begin to get a glimpse of the movement of time but are too busy owning the world to pay it much attention. Those in their forties are feeling their power but getting nervous at the same time about losing it. Fifty-pluses, who used to be able to start thinking about retirement and planning long vacations, are wondering whether they should start a new career. Over sixties, who were not only over the hill briefly ago in our social history but ancient, aren't anymore. The definition of the hill has changed as our population gets older and retains competence longer. That means there are a lot more of us approaching the hill than ever before but still actively involved in life. No wonder there is confusion.

The movement of life through the new hill, wherever that may be, is tough for men but intense for women. Not only do we have to deal with the numbers but also with the physical and emotional storms that knock on our doors and enter even when not invited in. The passage through menopause used to be the entrance into old age. Not anymore. If you think that because your children are grown and out of the house, that you have put in the requisite number of years at your job, that your mortgage is finally paid up, you are going to have it easy, forget it. Life goes on post children, post period, post retirement, post everything up to your final breath. The only thing you can count on is that life changes and you will change with it.

My mother's generation spoke of the change of life, that time somewhere in middle age when a woman started having hot flashes and stopped having a period. Conception was unlikely, though occasionally a change-of-life baby would appear on the scene. Physical discomfort and emotional instability were more certain. Men rolled their eyes with any deviation from normal routine and assumed it was female troubles.

This time they were right, it was a female issue. Women would take to their beds, as the saying went, so as either not to inconvenience anyone else with their complaints or to preserve decorum. More likely it was to prevent people knowing what they were experiencing because in a time when women were closely defined by their role in childbearing, cessation of that function was not welcome news. Menopause implied that real life was over for women, that everything past a certain age was irrelevant, including and especially them. No wonder so many women grew up dreading "the change" and did whatever they could to deny it.

That was then. Today, women talk about the changes their bodies are going through as openly as our mothers discussed the price of peas and toilet paper. It is a numbers thing. There are so many of us that menopause is often the topic of choice in any group. But the change-of-life stigma is as obsolete as women having the vapors.

There are changes, to be sure. No one is denying that. After all, we are modern women. We just handle it all differently. Our mothers wore aprons; we wear sweats. Our mothers didn't talk about personal matters; we tell all, to anyone, anywhere, often on the cell phone in the most crowded places. I have heard the most intimate conversations while standing on line at the post office, strap hanging on the bus, and trying to remain inconspicuous in the jury pool. Our mothers became matrons; we throw away our tampons and go dancing. Definitely, there are changes.

My sister went through menopause in her forties, as did my mother. My body waited until a decade later but the message was the same; you are taking a journey that every woman must take.

It is an odd journey because we often don't know when it begins and are surprised to discover we are already on it. At sixty-five, my mother-in-law said that she didn't know how she had gotten there but inside she felt thirty-five. I was thirty-three when she offered that little view into aging. I wondered, with all the smugness of someone who still saw life stretching on forever, how she could possibly feel my age. I never considered that she was still vital and active, that the nine organizations she belonged to had meaning other than to keep her busy. I looked past her vibrant attitude, ignored her physical beauty, and allowed my age prejudice to color the picture I was seeing. I could not project myself three decades later, nor was I willing to think about the changes that would someday alter my own life.

As the years advance for me, I understand what she meant. I stopped feeling my chronological age around forty-five. There was too much going on to be concerned with the wrinkles that began to appear. It was easy enough to pluck out the occasional gray hair that sprang up overnight and to moisturize the fine lines around my eyes. I could still laugh when I would forget a word and glibly call the lapse a senior moment without worrying about what might be coming.

I wasn't fooling the timekeeper, however. The lines got deeper and the gray spread as I moved into my fifties. Body parts started feeling the gravitational tug downward. There was definitely a shift in my time awareness. In one sense, though, I began to feel like a teenager again, experiencing menstrual cramps and mood swings. And then that changed into other manifestations of this midlife transition.

I had come to the hill with its new pathways and challenges. Like it or not, I would climb it, though not the way my mother's generation had. The isolation is gone. My friends are climbing with me. We share our experiences, laugh when we can and offer advice when needed. We live our lives the best we can, fighting the changes and accepting them at the same time, wondering where the time has gone and simultaneously seeing things with wonder from this new awareness.

The Adventures of Swamp Woman came about through this sharing. The book, through its personal essays, speaks to the transitions we are experiencing, sometimes gracefully but often fiercely. It reflects back to our beginnings and looks at where midlife is taking us. It is an ongoing conversation I am having with my friends, with my sister, and with the millions of sisters of my extended family, a conversation that extends along the continuum of the incredible experience called womanhood.

Transitions

Menopause Talking

I held the results of my latest DEXA Scan in my hand and they were not good. It revealed that I have osteopenia, a thinning of the bones that is on the way to being osteoporosis.

Three years ago I didn't even know what a DEXA Scan was. Now I was all too familiar with this x-ray of a person's bone density. Or in my case, the lack of density. The less dense bones become, the more likely a fracture. It could come from stepping wrong or turning sharply, a twisted ankle or a fall.

As I looked at the numbers, that old children's chant popped into my head: Step on a crack, break your mother's back. I remember carefully avoiding sidewalk cracks so that my mother's poor back wouldn't be in danger. Only, at this stage in my life, it's my back I am worried about.

When I whine to a friend about my bones, she tells me, "It's menopause talking."

I didn't know menopause had a voice. But my friend, who has gone through it and has perspective on this particular life transition, assures me that it does, indeed, speak. And it has a lot to say. I just have to listen.

I tell her whatever menopause wants to say to me, I don't want to hear it. But my unwillingness to have this conversation has not stopped menopause from piping in anyway. It comes unbidden and chatters away.

I have plenty of opportunity to listen to menopause in the early morning hours. For months I have been waking up every hour or so from two o'clock on until dawn.

True, I am able to get a lot of writing done during those peaceful hours when sleep is a stranger. And meditating as the sun smiles its good morning is quite lovely. Still, some quality sleep time would be welcome.

When I am rushing around, menopause whispers in my ear to slow down. "Take it easy," it says. "Take notice of your body's new needs and stop using it as a workhorse. Things are changing. Your body's timing is different now. You might want to rethink your productive hours and your rest times, perhaps take a midafternoon nap. After all, you really didn't get enough sleep last night, did you?"

I tell it I don't want to take a nap and I am not ready to slow down. I want to go exploring in the jungles of Malaysia. I want to go careening off-road in search of leopards in Africa and dogsledding in Alaska, all of which I've done in the past and might well do again. I am not ready to become menopause's partner. I notice, though, that I do enjoy a leisurely afternoon cup of tea.

I started to lift weights when my mother developed osteoporosis because I knew that weight-bearing exercise helped build bone density. I did it lip service, though, not really expecting to face this issue until I was well into my seventies, like Mom.

4

Yet here in my fifties, menopause is challenging me to be proactive in my health care. It says I have been playing with my training even though I lift heavier weights than some of the twenties who come to my gym. It is time to get stronger, to stimulate my bones into rebuilding themselves. Probably my mother had been getting messages about her bones, too, but either didn't listen or couldn't hear them. Maybe she just didn't know what to do.

I think I am finally getting it. I don't have to embrace menopause, just give it the respect it's due. After all, it is only me talking to myself. Now when I find myself ranting, I know it is menopause talking, telling me my chemistry is shifting. Time to take a deep breath. When my body temperature skyrockets, it reminds me that I am going through a profound transition and it shifts my focus to examining where I might be headed.

Perhaps this transition is leading me to greater self-awareness, although I seem to be going into it with all the grace of a charging rhino. I wonder if I am on the way to becoming a crone, one of those respected older wise women of other ages. Did they take everything in stride as they moved through their life transitions? Or did they, like me, question it all and resist until wisdom overtook them.

Did they hear menopause talking, too?

Yogurt Love

It was like that scene from the movie *When Harry Met Sally*. You know the one, where Sally fakes an orgasm at the restaurant table, moaning and shouting so convincingly that the woman at the next table tells the server she'll have the same thing. That was how I felt the second the spoon touched my lips. I melted. My whole body sang with sweetness and the cool caress of that exquisite taste. I felt my knees weaken and I had to sit down.

One might expect that reaction toward Godiva chocolate, say, or a perfectly baked caramel flan. This was neither. No, this was cherry vanilla yogurt straight out of a plastic cup. It was the first yogurt I'd had in my mouth for over ten years and I was in love.

This is not an easy thing for a vegan to admit. Vegans, after all, do not eat yogurt. Or any milk products. We don't eat eggs or fish. Certainly not poultry. Forget about meat. So what was I doing rhapsodizing about yogurt?

My sister said, "Look what you've been missing." My friend said, "Why did you deprive yourself for so long?"

Neither comment had any relevance. I did not feel that I was missing anything nor did I feel deprived in any way. I have been vegetarian for almost thirty years and vegan for eleven so this was not some crazy diet, as my father once called it. I was acting on my philosophy. And that is what makes shifting so difficult for me. Not only am I changing what I eat but how I think. More than that, I am redefining who I am. At the very least, I am someone who is no longer vegan.

My bones are the cause of all this. They are getting thinner. Not that I feel it yet. I have not shrunk and I am stronger than ever. No one would suspect that my bones are being resorbed. But the DEXA Scan knows. It is clear on the X-ray. In this case, the numbers don't lie. It is a clarion call to pay attention to my body.

I can't pretend that what worked for me in my earlier adult years is appropriate now. It isn't. I need to work with my philosophy to come to an understanding about my whole being, body included, at this time in my life, which is different from any other time I have experienced.

There is no way that I can ignore this body/ philosophy conversation. My philosophy says that I do not eat conscious creatures or their products. My body says that I am doing it harm by not considering a shift in thinking. My philosophy says that vegetarianism is an honored spiritual choice. My body says each being has its own needs. My philosophy says that I don't want to abandon my principles. My body says it will still respect me in the morning.

I consulted an ayuruvedic practitioner. Ayurveda is the Hindu science of life through a nutritional perspective. She confirmed what my body was telling me. And added my need for more protein as well. Soy was good but not cutting it for me. Knowing that I have three definite risk factors already (small frame, fair skin and heredity) for osteoporosis, I thought that I would reexamine my beliefs in regard to food. What it came down to was my respect for all life. Could I eat higher up on the food chain and take care of my new bodily needs, at the same time maintaining this philosophy? Would I be compromising my spirit by doing so? Would I be disrespectful to my gift of life to disregard what my bones were telling me? Could I be as nonjudgmental with myself as I profess to be with others?

I decided on a balance. I would eat the dairy products that were good for me because my body needed them but would stay away from those that would clog my system and cause other issues. I would eat fish as well as soy to step up the regeneration of my body but I would do it with consciousness. A life given for a life deserves that much. And considering that I believe that all of creation is conscious on some level, I would try to eat deliberately, not automatically.

This has been welcome news for everyone around me. My husband says it is grand to be able to once again enjoy the same dinner with me. I have been making separate meals or variations on a vegetarian theme for three decades. My friend said that it has opened up new possibilities for when I visit. Cooking for me had been for her what she politely called a pain in the pan.

They easily embraced the new me. I am still exploring, day by day, who I am. I have to go with the broadest aspect of my philosophy, which is to be flexible. Sometimes our greatest growth comes where we least expect to find it. A cup of yogurt is hardly the stuff songs are written about, but it inspired in me an internal dialogue and an appreciation for the interaction of all the parts that make up a human being. The care of each is essential to the optimal functioning of the whole. Today I love yogurt, but who knows what my body will tell me tomorrow. I wonder if there is a hot fudge sundae in my future.

Living in the Hot Lane

I feel it approaching, the way you know when a train is about to hit the station before you see it. Two seconds later it comes roaring in, the ol' hot flash express, filling me with its suddenness, its engine steaming inside me. I hope it will pass through quickly and I'll be able to get on with what I am doing. If not, I will have to carry on anyway. Life doesn't stop just because I'm living in the hot lane.

I have tried to describe what a hot flash feels like to my husband but there is really no way he can know without experiencing it. What he does feel is the outer manifestation. He says I am swampy. He is right. Rivulets of sweat flow down my body, pooling in any small indentation: the crook of an elbow, back of my knees, between my breasts. I have a friend who loves hot weather, the hotter the better, yet she said that on the hottest day she never felt as hot as she did when she was flashing. She complained that her ankles sweat. She is past flashing now and empathizes with me but she doesn't miss it.

I am grateful that I work at home. I can get up from my computer and jump into the tub when it gets too uncomfortable. I don't have to worry about leaving a puddle on my chair at an important client's meeting.

I have been known to stick my head inside the freezer when it really gets to me.

One friend who does go to client meetings never lets on when she is burning up. She has, however, allowed her hair to grow a little longer so she can cover her ears. They turn bright pink when she flashes.

Another friend is also experiencing this transition. Her husband says that she turns the air conditioner so low at night, he has icicles forming in his nostrils.

It suddenly makes sense to me why men and women had separate bedrooms in former times. It wasn't because of modesty or the need for privacy. It was temperature control. She wanted the windows open; he wanted them closed.

The standard advice for flashers is to take hormone replacement therapy. But it is not for everyone. Not for my friend with a heart condition, or for the one with a family history of ovarian cancer. Not for me with my alternative philosophy. And since research has shown that HRT actually increases the risk of heart disease, cancer, blood clots and stroke, many more women are looking for other options.

So we balance wild yam and soy, primrose oil and dong quai, looking for the combinations that work for us. And we talk to each other, sharing our stories and laughing. One thing we discovered is that none of us feel our femininity is threatened by the knowledge that one day soon we will not be able to have children, once a common worry of menopausal women. Our sex drive is still in gear though it may be in second instead of fifth.

This isn't a disease that needs to be cured. It is just a natural part of the maturing process. Some of us feel it more acutely than others but we are individuals and bound to vary in our responses to this time of life.

We don't deny what we are going through, we work through it with information and accommodation and intelligence.

What we have noticed is that our sisterhood has deepened. We cannot talk about such intimate things without drawing closer. And that has many benefits. We see how we have grown over the years because we are no longer afraid or embarrassed to tell the truth. With truth comes power. We know who we are now. We accept ourselves with all the flaws and inconsistencies that come with living actively. At least most of the time. When we have doubts, we go to each other knowing there will be a receptive ear and no judgment.

So what if living in the hot lane has its inconveniences? They will pass eventually but the joy we women have in each other will remain. We are getting the better of the deal.

Where Are the Cookies?

"Where are the cookies?" my husband asks, his head deep in the pantry.

"Not there," I answer.

"The candy? The chocolate bits? Where is anything to eat that isn't good for you?" he grumbles.

As I grope my way through change-of-life issues, he is learning to cope with change-of-pantry withdrawal. Legions of vitamins and herbs and shelves of tea have replaced the cans of condensed soup, packages of cookies, and boxes of macaroni and cheese. Sugared cereals have given way to granola, candy bars to multigrain bread. Everything is calcium enriched and isoflavone enhanced.

Part of this change comes from a general societal shift that recognizes the importance of good nutrition. Cookies are not suggested in any of the major food groups, and the sodium content in most canned soups would give pause to the cows at the salt lick. Part of it is a search for a more natural way of eating, free of preservatives and trans fats. Still another part comes from the ecological awareness of limiting excess packaging. All great reasons for stocking up on fiber contained in whole grains and minimally processed foods.

But I must be truthful. The main reason for the pantry alteration is to accommodate the needs of this new life stage I'm going through. My body is shifting. Foods I used to eat without a second thought have turned against me. Sugar gives me headaches. Chocolate sets up cravings that wipe out any idea of real food. Unrefined carbs go straight to my waist and after doing their damage disappear in a New York minute leaving me with a ravenous hunger and a calorie intake more attuned to a sumo wrestler than to a small, midlife female.

This is all anecdotal observation. Noticeable patterns. Other women may experience different responses to the same foods. I make this disclaimer because we have been weaned on the scientific method. Science tends to pooh-pooh anecdotal evidence but since billions of dollars are being spent each year on health foods and nutritional supplements, propelled in good part by menopausal women, there has been a new emphasis on women's needs. The almost exclusively male model of medicine and nutrition has broken down. Science has discovered there is money to be made from women! Vitamins, minerals and herbs are the hot (no pun intended) medical topics.

So my pantry is well stocked with Vitamins A, C and E for their antioxidant value. Calcium and magnesium tablets for strong bones are cozily nestled next to dong quai and black cohosh, which regulate the hormones. Evening primrose capsules and red clover chase away the hot flashes. Raspberry leaf tea regulates the estrogenic cycle (what's left of it), peppermint tea aids in digestion and green tea from China and Japan guards against cancer. I am thankful to all these supplements for keeping me healthy because there is no room in on my shelves for anything the drug companies have to offer. Or for cookies.

My husband grumbles as he burrows behind the containers of soy milk, dried fruit and protein bars, digging further into the pantry looking for something appetizing.

"Have some chips," I suggest.

"We have chips?"

He reaches for the non-aluminum lined bags to discover taro, baked not fried corn, sesame-soy and sweet potato chips.

"We don't have chips," he says as he puts the bags back on the shelf. "We don't have anything edible!" he wails.

"Keep looking," I tell him.

He finally comes up with one of the shiny, crackly, jiggly bags of double chocolate chips I buy especially for him. His face lights up as he tears into it and pops the chunky chocolate bits into his mouth, savoring each one as it melts on his tongue.

I may be health conscious and I may be menopausal but I am not cruel. Sometimes a man just needs his chocolate the way a woman needs her soy. My pantry knows it. And so do I.

The Squeaky Wheel

I remember my mother saying to my grandmother when I was young and acting up, "The squeaky wheel gets the oil." Then she would hand me a cookie or a slap whichever she felt was appropriate.

I hadn't understood what she meant back then. I wasn't a wheel. I shouted, cried, laughed, and occasionally talked back but I didn't squeak. All I knew was that for better or worse, acting up got her attention.

Now that I'm well grown up, I find myself revisiting that squeaky wheel concept from a different perspective. I may still not be a wheel but I sure am squeaky. At least my joints are. Every bend, every knuckle, every possible place that can crack or creak or squeak does. My shoulder cricks when I lift the barbell during my gym workout. My elbow cracks when I open the door. My ankles set up a percussion riff as I walk and my knees could substitute for the starting gun at the Boston marathon.

So, in lieu of cookies and gratefully instead of a slap, I now take my mother's saying literally and give all my squeaks the oil and attention that they require. More oil goes on my body than in it.

My husband knows which oil I am using for my daily massage by the aromas that waft through the house.

"Chinese food today?" he asks when I slather on the sesame oil.

Sometimes the house is redolent of coconut oil and the south pacific islands. Olive oil brings the aroma of the ripe Italian countryside. Often the house picks up a mixture of several scents, creating a world fusion atmosphere. It is somewhat disconcerting to have this heady brew assault your nostrils at seven in the morning but the squeaky wheel…

I am amazed that my body has become so vocal, and I often find it embarrassing. Once my trainer at the gym was worried that I broke something because the crack was so loud. No, I assured him, it's just my elbow telling him what it thought of his regimen.

In the senior stretching class I run at an assisted living residence, I am the only one whose body talks. I am at least twenty years younger than any of them and no one's joints creak except mine.

"Listen to her bones," they chuckle. "Maybe she should move in here with us."

I laugh with them and make jokes at my own expense but I am not happy about the situation. My body moves fine, thank goodness, and has no particular limitations. When I look at all the ailments in front of me, I am grateful that all I have to deal with is noise.

But I don't understand how my body can work so well and sound so bad. Is it age asserting its newfound power? Is arthritis testing itself against my determination to keep flexible? Can I blame hormones, because it's so easy to lay any complaint at that cause?

Perhaps it's just my body's way of reminding me to pay it some attention.

So I pour on the oil. My skin feels wonderfully soft but the squeaks have not stopped. I have added taking omega −3 capsules. Oil outside, oil inside. And I am still the squeaky wheel.

Maybe I am making too much of this. What does it matter if I have this dialogue going with my own body? As long as I am healthy and happy, a little creakiness shouldn't spoil things. I am, after all, living the life I choose and I am grateful. No one stops me from having my say. Not since I was a little girl acting up. If all my joints want to speak up, who am I to grumble about it?

Thank you, body, for supporting me so beautifully.

Here, have a cookie and squeak on.

Yo Yo Ma

I am speaking to my daughter. I try to be perky but after another night of broken sleep, my weariness comes across the phone lines. She hears it.

"What's wrong?" she asks.

"I'm tired," I tell her. "I don't sleep well. I fall asleep fine but then I wake up a few hours later. I go back to sleep and wake up. Sleep and wake up. All through the night. I'm pooped."

"You sound like a yo-yo, Ma."

I feel like one. Up and down all night. I haven't had a good night's sleep in two years, ever since I started menopause.

I knew about hot flashes and irritability, headaches and bone loss. Sleep disturbance was a surprise to me although it is one of the classic symptoms. There is an actual pattern to it. Something, often a sound, triggers a rush of adrenalin, which stresses the adrenals which causes a hot flash which initiates sweating which leads to a cooling of the body and bone chattering chills. Then the cycle starts over again, picking up speed as the night progresses because the adrenal glands become more stressed and respond to smaller triggers.

After the first few months, it was easy to discover the rhythm. To me the process resembles a well-orchestrated symphony in which I am playing all the instruments. The night's overture introduces the main theme of sleeping and waking. Then the Temperature Variations arise. One movement has me surging with heat in a crescendo that drags me from the deepest sleep to a fully awakened state with every pore in my body open and sweating in fortissimo. I throw off the covers and seek each cool spot on the sheet. This shifts into the next movement where the intensity relaxes and I drift off into an adagio of dreams. That leads into an expressive scherzo as I once again awaken, this time in a freezing counterpoint, and scramble for the covers, pulling them up to my chin to ease the shivering. The symphony ends with a spirited sleeping and awakening rondo of increasing tempo that ends with the click of the clock radio announcing the beginning of another active day.

I hope I am up to it.

There are ways to modify the disturbance. A glass of warm milk at bedtime. Lavender in the bathtub. Soothing visualization to relax the whole system. An infusion of nettle tea to calm the adrenals. An occasional shot of valerian root. They all work sometimes and don't at other times. It is frequently tempting to try all of them at once but I would be so busy infusing and bathing and fantasizing and gulping that I probably wouldn't get any more sleep than had I not done anything.

Besides, there is a certain perverse comfort in the predictability of it all. I don't have to look at the clock to know that it is two in the morning. There is peace in the house then and I can appreciate the silence. Part of the enjoyment of going to a familiar concert is to anticipate each musical phrase.

Despite the beauty of the nightly performance, however, I admit that I wouldn't mind sleeping through it. Barring that, perhaps I should get out of bed when I wake up the first time. I would at least have the extra time to accomplish something useful instead of churning the bed sheets. Like writing the Great American Novel. I would probably have enough time to write the Great Russian Novel.

I might go back to painting and create a whole new school of art. I could call it Menopaulism. It would reflect the convergence of the altered perception that emerges from the sleep-deprived state with the cosmic expression of female empowerment. Sort of Timothy Leary on hormones.

Maybe I'll just forget about sleeping altogether and take up the cello.

The Adventures of Swamp Woman

"I think I'll start wearing scuba gear to bed," my husband said the other night. "I don't want to drown."

"Ha Ha," I replied. But I could sympathize. I wish I could protect myself from myself. Hardly a night passes where I am not awakened awash in steamy sweat. I have turned into Swamp Woman. It is the Curse of the Crone.

That would make a great title for a horror movie. Let's see. Swamp Woman is a perfectly normal person until her mid-fifties when she suddenly straps on a backpack and goes trekking in Borneo. There she barely escapes being dragged out of a longboat by a rabid crocodile but not before she is injected with the jungle virus through the crocodile's bite, and now, each night, she becomes an oozing creature of the jungle waters looking for relief. She turns first to her family for support, nearly drowning her husband in a hug when all she really wants to do is assure herself that she is still desirable. She slimes her way to her children's bedrooms, hoping to get the help she needs, but cannot find a single dry towel. In her mad, wet resolve, she vows to experiment until she discovers the herbs that will ease the heat raging inside her. She uses her friends as test subjects and leaves a trail of chemically altered mutants behind her.

I haven't figured out the ending yet, but just think of the possibilities for special effects. We could leave out the part that menopause plays in this; it's much better fictionalized.

Menopause has brought out in me a whole host of skills I never knew I possessed. Besides dreaming up screenplays, I am now a fashion consultant for my friends who are shifting into the wet season. We choose clothes by how little they show the damp spots. Black is the preferred color. Twins sets are good because the outer sweater can be removed when the heat rises and then popped back on when the under sweater soaks through and the chills start. Beading is concealing on fancy wear and a shawl adds just the right fashion touch, especially when shoulders begin to dissolve atop a slinky evening gown.

I have become a stress counselor for women's groups, offering understanding and techniques to those who are experiencing the transition into mature womanhood and need help coping. My years of yoga have at last come in handy. Breathe, I tell them. Focus. Find your inner puddle, I mean your core. These workshops have a de-stressing effect on me as well once I get going, but I must admit that planning for them makes me nervous enough to have flash attacks beforehand.

My mother never prepared me for this. Back then women didn't talk about such things. They endured in silence or threw tantrums but did not reveal the source of their distress. In all fairness, maybe my mother didn't have hot flashes. Not every woman does. Somewhere between fifty percent and eighty-five percent of women experience hot flashes and night sweats. That means a lucky fifty percent to fifteen percent escape with their internal thermometer intact.

My daughter won't be able to say that about me. She has seen me turn scarlet over the salad course at a restaurant. She has watched her mother prance around in a T-shirt and shorts during a winter freeze when she, herself, was sitting in the kitchen wearing a hat and scarf. She knows what is going on. She reminds me to breathe.

I think it is important to share the full life cycle. Let my daughter see how I deal with maturing. It will give her something to laugh about when she is in the same position, if she is, and maybe offer some insights into the joys and challenges that come with female aging.

And there are joys. Like knowing who you are, at last. Like having the freedom to explore parts of yourself that were kept in check by the responsibilities of youth and middle age. Appreciating the resonance of long-time friendships. Feeling the throb of life within the changes going on.

So, back to the adventures of Swamp Woman. We last saw her experimenting in the laboratory looking for the precise combination of ingredients to halt the insidious creeping night sweats. She has been reading about cooling substances from the annals of herbalism, ayurveda and traditional Chinese medicine. She brews a mixture of black cohosh, basil, coconut oil, dried peaches and rose buds. She cools the bubbling mixture, then purees and strains it into a glass. It looks like toxic sludge but to Swamp Woman it represents hope. Now for the test. Does she drink it or slather it all over her body? The fire is stoking itself inside her like an alien being. Do it. Do it now! She holds up the glass. It is time.

The tension is unbearable. I think I'll sit quietly and do my breathing practice. And while I'm calm, maybe I can come up with further adventures: Flood and Fire in the Suburbs, The Revenge of Swamp Woman, or perhaps, and this is my personal favorite, Swamp Woman Out of Control. Who knows where this could lead. Perhaps I'll have a whole new career. I believe in seeing things in a positive light. When life hands out lemons, I'll be the first in line at the lemonade stand. More ice, please.

Video Views

Someone I was supposed to know said hello to me today. She looked familiar but for the life of me, I couldn't remember who she was. She certainly knew me. She referred to my children, by name, and inquired about their whereabouts. (Could she be a neighbor from the far side of my long street?) She asked if I was still writing children's books. (Was she someone I should know professionally?)

I answered her questions and wanted to ask about her current doings but unless I figured out how we connected, I had nothing to contribute to the conversation that wasn't weather talk, the generic babble that passes for polite chatter. Did she have children? I didn't know. So I took a deep breath and said, "Please remind me how I know you. My memory isn't what it used to be."

It turned out that she was someone I had worked with when we volunteered in our children's elementary school library. Ah, yes. It came back. I could see an inner picture of her at the library desk stamping out the books. A friendly person I had always liked. Her name came right to me at that moment. But until the inner picture appeared to place her in a context, I had no clue as to her identity.

I am finding that happening more often than I would care to admit. I don't know if it is memory loss or the fuzziness that comes from shifting hormones. Lack of concentration seems to be one of the symptoms of menopause.

I am not alone in this predicament. My sister once complained that she didn't recognize the nurse from her gynecologist's office when they met in a store. She had been seeing this woman twice a year for three decades but without the uniform and the familiar environment, there was no recognition.

My friends have various ways of handling their occasional memory lapses. One told me that faces are easy for her to remember but that names elude her. To compensate, she forms a silly image in her mind when she is introduced to someone new so she has something to connect with the name. Andy Barr might end up as a huge Snickers in her mind, a candy bar to remember Andy Barr. The more outrageous the image, the more memorable, she tells me. For some reason, she can remember the image and that leads her to the name.

Another friend said when she has trouble calling up someone's name, she runs through the alphabet in her head. The name usually pops into her mind when she gets to the beginning letter.

We are all playing mental name games. My particular game is viewing the subject as though I am panning through a video camera. It brings in the person and the surroundings which most of the time leads to my recalling the name before I awkwardly have to, as I did with my library co-worker, ask.

It works with other memory lapses, too. If I am trying to recall a word, I will see a scene that signifies its meaning. In trying to call up a species of tree, for instance, I may focus on a forest with many trees and zoom in on the leaf of the tree I want, which might bring the name of that specific tree into my head. Or not. I can't guarantee it will always work. Sometimes I end up with a beautifully blank field and no word at all.

This terrifies me. My mother had Alzheimer's disease so every lapse creates a scene of my mother's babbling. In this, I am also not alone. My sister, too, panics when she reaches for a word and can't grab it. Words have become her, and my, brass rings. Each word retrieved is a valuable prize. Many of our friends share this fear as they see their parents succumb to dementia. Alzheimer's is a generational scourge.

"Put me in a home by the sea," I tell my daughter. "At the first sign of goofiness."

"How will I know when that is?" she says. "You're pretty goofy now."

"When I'm goofier. When I start mistaking my electric toothbrush for a cell phone. Or if you see me wearing my underwear for my outerwear."

"Don't I remember you wearing boxer shorts on your head one year when you were teaching yoga?"

"That was for educational purposes," I remind her. "I was talking to my class about being flexible and enjoying life."

"How about the dryer lint you shaped into bugs and hung over the doorway? That was pretty goofy, I'd say."

"I was trying out a Halloween activity for a kids' book!"

"So that doesn't count as evidence for putting you in a home?"

"No, not yet. But when I do that stuff without a purpose, that's the right time. You don't even have to come and visit. In fact, don't visit. I won't know you anyway. I'll be happy dribbling soup down my shirt and listening to the waves. Of course, I probably won't know what waves are any more, either, but that's okay. I like the shore."

She assures me that she will take care of me no matter what. But I don't want her to have to care for me. When she was a teen, my daughter and her friends used to ask each other, "Which would you rather be, blind or deaf? Would you rather lose a leg or an arm?" They were exploring different interactions with their world. I ask myself now, which would I rather have, a long life with Alzheimer's or a short life with my mental faculties intact? There is no philosophical angst for me. I'd rather be outta here.

I try to assure myself that my current memory issues are within the normal range of aging behaviors. My father, who is in his late eighties, tells me he doesn't remember any of the trips he had taken. Even with photographs to prompt him, the connections are gone. But he doesn't have Alzheimer's.

Stress wreaks havoc with everyone's memory and there is more than an acceptable amount of that in this world of terrorists blowing themselves up and taking a host of innocent people with them.

Some people work well under pressure. I don't. As a child, I was never very good at coming up with the right answer when the teacher called on me in class. So why should it be different for me now when I'm confronted with a situation that demands immediate recognition? And with my hormones playing a game of marbles (assuming, of course I am not losing mine) in my system, that can only make instant memory a more iffy proposition.

The panic abates when I think of this. Until I grope for another word. Then I rely on my mental video camera to bring my memory into focus. I adjust the lens to sharpen the image and hope for the best. If the image doesn't bring the word into my head, at least I can console myself that I'm not yet material for the home. I still use my toothbrush to clean my teeth.

Through the Lens

I had my photo taken recently. It was a head shot for a magazine. I have lots of photos of me on trips and with family but I hadn't taken a straight-on close-up in a long time. When I saw the picture, it was something of a surprise. I looked tired even though I wasn't at the time. My almond eyes, once my most exquisite physical feature, had tiny suitcases beneath them. My eyelids drooped so that my eyes more resembled the slits of a prowling stray cat than the enchanting eyes of Nefertiti, to which they were once compared. And although I knew my hair was gray because of a conscious decision on my part not to dye it, it was grayer than I realized.

Do I really look like that? I wondered. But photographs don't lie, do they?

I had always laughed at the youthful photos on book jackets when everyone knew the author was four hundred years old. Who were they kidding? We readers know the truth. Let us see how they really look at the age they wrote the book. We can take it. Yet now with the tables turned, could I take it?

It distressed me to think that the photo would be all that readers would know about me. It reflected such a small part of who I am. Would anyone looking at it see the person who rode an elephant in Africa or supported a friend during her bout with cancer? Was it obvious that I love to dance or that I write books for children? Could anyone know from that photo that I meditate and do tai chi and lift weights? What distressed me most, however, was that I was even asking myself those questions.

I knew what prompted this face-to-face confrontation. A few days before I met someone I hadn't seen since my children were in elementary school. She looked pretty much the same except that now her hair was creamy brown instead of the salt and pepper it was becoming back then. It threw me into retro-thought. I used to have brown hair. I used to be the mother of young children. I was twenty once and thirty and had years ahead to think about such trivial stuff as wrinkles and gray hair. The idea of droopy eyelids or skin like a worn-out rubber band was something I couldn't have imagined. On me. Ever.

I used to have the kind of face that looked years younger. People were always amazed that I had two children and marveled at their ages. Lately, no one has shown surprise when they find out how old I am or that my children are grown. The photo clarified why. I look the way I am supposed to look at my age.

I considered going the facelift route until I watched a documentary about it on television and saw the plastic surgeon peel off the patient's face. It was too gross to contemplate. I know there is no way that I will be able to do it. I get queasy from a paper cut. I once almost fainted just having a mole removed. What would I do if my whole face were relocated? The mere thought of the procedure would have me losing my lunch, which will not exactly enhance my appearance.

I stared hard at that photo. What was so terrible about my not looking like a starlet? I never did when I was younger, why should I expect to now? What, exactly, did I see? I saw myself as I was. And my self seemed to say that was okay.

There is a time for everything in life. This is the time for me to step up and declare my independence from the fashion magazine image of beauty, to claim the radiance that is evident from within.

I will revamp my whole way of thinking. Instead of crow's feet, I plan to think of the fine wrinkles around my eyes as crone's pleats, the fabric of wisdom that comes with living an eventful life. The bags under my eyes I shall choose to see as reflective of a mind too active to get the proper rest. And the gray hair that miraculously weaves a head of ordinary brown strands with silver chains that glint in the sunlight I will associate with the ripening of the spirit, like the leaves of autumn that display their true colors only after the green of youth has faded.

Now that I have all of this obvious wisdom, I intend to use it in a practical way. To find the best moisturizers that modern science has come up with. To gather the finest rejuvenating herbs of ancient knowledge. To explore every holistic practice that detoxifies and revitalizes. Because a wise person knows that the present is all that is given to any of us. That photograph is my present.

And while I appreciate the crone I one day hope to be, I will leave the future to some other photo and work with what I have now.

Mirror Image

There I was, staring into the bedroom mirror wondering what was wrong. The image staring back was obviously me but not quite. Something was definitely out of whack.

Then it hit me. The mirror was lying. The whole premise of a mirror is falsehood. A mirror's nature is to show the opposite of what is actually facing it. Touch your right ear while facing a mirror and the image touches its left ear. Point over there at the image and the image points back here at you. How can you believe a mirror?

So when the mirror showed me as a woman in her fifties, it was clearly is a distortion of what is real. The age I feel is not a day over thirty-something. Now that I know the nature of the mirror, that right is left and there is really here, older must actually mean younger. Then that poochie stomach the mirror presents me with must mean that the stomach on the real me is nicely tucked in. Out and in are opposites, after all.

People have called me naïve. Now I know why. I could so easily be fooled by an inanimate silvered object.

I also used to think that photographs didn't lie. What they showed was reality. Yes, I knew about airbrushing out unwanted lines but for the most part, a photo was a document that could be trusted. Now, in the digital age, I wouldn't trust a photo further than I could throw a flatbed scanner. It can be digitally manipulated to show anything the photographer has in mind. Digital photography is a brushstroke (or an icon) away from a painting. What eluded me for the longest time, however, was that a camera was really a mirror and so, of course, the photographic image that resulted from a picture being taken had to lie.

Since becoming aware of the mirror principle of opposites, I am beginning to see the influence of these perverse images all around me.

In my gym, there is a machine with a shiny convex surface that makes whoever is staring into it look elongated, happy and delightfully fit. I would hardly compare my five-foot-two body to a Modigliani figure. Nor would I describe myself as happy when I am pitting myself against a fifty-pound weight and grunting. The smile reflected on the machine is actually a grimace. Opposites, again. I see an image that shows my muscles popping and the buffest bod in the place. Unfortunately, this is a mirror so it must be showing the reverse of reality, which means I have a lot more work to do if I want to tone up my muscles. It is great motivation, however. I want to look like that image. So I keep at it because that reflected bod must be possible. When I see a flabby, frowning gnome glowering back at me, I will know that all my efforts have finally resulted in success.

This is not the only example of mirror distortion.

What about the side view mirror on the right of the car? It shows an image of the car behind or on the side. It seems to be reasonably far away so it should be safe for changing lanes. Isn't it there to make driving safer?

Only there is a little notice right there on the mirror that says that the image is closer than it appears. It shows it far but it really is near. Another mirror lie.

Look straight into a telescope in a conservatory and see planets and stars. But it is only a trick of many mirrors angled this way and that that allows the light images to be observed. The problem is that if we can see the light it is already gone. Light here, light not there. We are seeing phantoms.

And what about the eyeball? It isn't officially a mirror but it might as well be. A lens takes in optical information and flips it upside down. Without that image being interpreted and repositioned by the brain, we would all be walking around on our heads, trying to make sense of the opposites we were seeing.

But maybe that is the key. The old saying, Beauty is in the eye of the beholder, really should say, Beauty is in the mind of the beholder. We see things upside down but interpret them right side up. Mirrors show us opposites but we understand them to be the reverse of what we see.

So I think I'll pull a mirror and think the opposite.

I can focus on a flabby tummy and worry about my shape or see that I am in good health and be glad, depending on how I interpret what the mirror shows.

I can find wrinkles and groan about it or discover new character reflected in my face.

I can see fifty and still feel thirty.

After all, it isn't the mirror's job to interpret its reflection. It is up to us to see the good, the bad, and the beautiful.

Touch-up Touchy

I'm beginning to feel touchy about my hair being gray. When my aunt complimented me on the nubby gray sweater I was wearing by asking me where on earth I was able to find a sweater to match my hair so perfectly, I seriously thought of going out and dying my hair.

That may have been the most blatant comment but there have been lots of others recently that seemed to me to be oblique references to my gray tresses. There was the time when the cashier in the supermarket asked me if I needed help with my grocery bags. I might have overlooked it as mere politeness except that my older sister, who highlights her hair blonde and shops in the same market, was not asked that particular question.

Once, in the shopping mall, a fresh-faced young kiosk person made a beeline over to me as I exited a store. "I can tell you're a natural woman," she said. Then she proceeded to make a pitch for some nail product that would smooth out the ridges in my nails and make them beautiful. I was flattered that she realized I am not one for ostentation, an easy call as I was wearing my gym clothes and not a bit of jewelry. But the product did address an issue I was having with my nails so I bought it. As I was leaving, I noticed that she accosted another woman with the same line. This woman wore enough jangling jewelry to hold a concert by herself and was dressed from the Nieman Marcus catalogue. The only similarity between us was our gray hair.

And just this very week, a clerk in a department store asked me if I was the one who put aside a package to be picked up later. I assured her that I was not but she kept insisting, insinuating that I was wrong and did, indeed, leave that package there.

"She looked like you," the clerk said.

"She's some other woman with gray hair," I said testily as she rang up my purchases. I left the store before she had the idea to ask if I qualified for the senior discount, in which case I would have immediately sent in my Extreme Makeover video.

"You're getting too sensitive about this," my sister said. "If it bothers you that much, why don't you touch up the gray?"

But I won't do it for a number of reasons. I know me. I am lazy. I'll be lax about making appointments at the hairdresser so I'll have gray peeking through anyway, defeating my purpose. Or if I do it on my own, I'll end up with multicolored patches on my scalp that will make me look like a circus clown because I'll forget which hair product I used last time and each company has its own spectrum. But mainly, I don't like the idea of putting chemicals on my head. I use all-natural shampoos (the mall woman was right there) and would get creeped out thinking of the stuff that was leeching into my brain.

I actually don't mind my hair color. It is more a silver than battleship gray. Quite becoming, I think. I just don't want it to be the first or the only thing people notice about me. I don't want to be a victim of hairism, having assumptions made about me based on my hair color.

Today, when the supermarket cashier asked me again if I needed help out with my packages, I knew I had to say something.

"Why did you ask me that? Is it because I have gray hair?"

She pointed to my cart. "We're supposed to ask anyone who has more than two grocery bags if they want help. It's policy. Sometimes we forget but we're really supposed to ask."

"Oh," I said. There were six full bags in my cart, bags bursting with melons and crusty breads, overflowing with bright robust carrots, rainbow chard, and wispy sprays of dill. All were heavy with the delicious goods the store offered.

"Well, thank you but no, I don't need help," I said and slunk out of the store feeling foolish. I had created my own insult where none existed.

Maybe my sister is right and I am being a bit touchy. I think I'll take her advice and get a touch-up. But it will be my attitude, not my hair, that gets the attention.

The Power of Being Dishy

I was in a dress store making my first foray at mother-of-the-groom dresses. My son propelled me into this category by announcing he was getting married. I was delighted to hear the news. I love his fiancée and see a great future for them. My husband and I even get along well with her parents and the rest of her family. So, with a late winter wedding in mind, I started to browse in the specialty shops for styles that would be pretty and appropriate for my fifty-six years and my new role. I had no intention of purchasing anything until three or four months down the road. After all, the bride-to-be hadn't yet bought her gown. Knowing that I wasn't buying freed me to try on whatever caught my eye.

All that was forgotten when I tried on The Dress. Why this one called to me, at this time in my life, I'll never know. It was strapless with a beaded bodice and a long, softly flowing skirt. I thought I looked good in it in the dressing room but I have been known to pick out clothes that were less than flattering. I tend toward folksy styles with so much material that my thin frame sometimes gets lost. When I came out to show the salesperson, however, I knew it was right. There were eight people in the shop and eight pairs of eyes lit up. Nine, if you counted mine. I had never worn a strapless dress before. I never thought I could carry it off. I was carrying this dress like I was born to wear it.

"That dress looks great on you," said one of the other customers. "You have the shoulders for it."

My trainer at the gym would be happy to hear it.

An older gentleman who was waiting sleepily in a chair while his wife tried on one dress after another was suddenly alert. He didn't say a word but he didn't have to. I could tell I looked sexy. I felt sexy. His wife was trying on a more traditional style dress and jacket, more like what I had expected to look at and for a moment I had a twinge of doubt. She was older by a good fifteen years but we had the same amount of gray hair. Was I being foolish? She looked at me with a discerning eye, appraised me as I stood not four feet from her, and smiled. I smiled shyly back in appreciation.

"This dress fits you like a glove," said the salesperson. "Usually we have to take in a few tucks here and there but not this time."

I preened in front of the three-way mirror a little while longer before deciding to buy the dress. How could I not? One doesn't turn down Cinderella's gown. I walked out of the shop feeling like royalty.

I tried on the dress for my husband and got the same lit-up reaction.

"You look dishy," he said.

I laughed at the old-fashioned compliment and immediately became nervous. Was it okay for me to look dishy? Would it embarrass my son? Would it embarrass me? Was someone in her mid fifties supposed to look that way? And why did it feel so good?

I didn't think of myself as dishy as a teenager. My hair was too straight, my body too skinny and flat. I remember wishing that I would be sexy but when I developed curves, they seemed foreign so I covered them up. That did nothing to enhance my appeal. I was smart but didn't see the desirability of that at the time. Later on, I worked at being professional and efficient as a girl maturing during the feminist revolution would.

Now here I was, lapping up the admiring stares. I was glowing. But it was more about sensuality than sexuality. I didn't really care what was going through other people's heads when they saw me in the dress, though it was amusing to think that I might be prompting some lascivious thoughts. I just knew that I felt fluid and graceful.

I wasn't trying to return to my youth, an impossibility after two children and thirty-seven years of marriage. It wasn't necessary anyway. Dishyness is not a function of youth. I have a friend who is closer to seventy than fifty who has people of various ages flocking around her with that light in their eyes. She recognized her sensuality all along while I played hide and seek with it for five decades before finding it.

To my surprise, I enjoyed being dishy. This new perception of myself was fun. There was energy here, a power that radiated from me and was recognized by others. I started carrying myself differently. I walked taller and easier with the confidence of someone who has been a dish all of her life. I noticed that people smiled more at me but maybe that was because I found myself smiling more in general.

The dress helped me claim the sensuality I owned but never accepted. It did more for me than just provide me with a dress for this wonderful occasion. I knew I would look smashing. I was going to have a wonderful time at the wedding, too busy dancing to worry about my son, whose attention would be focused on his beautiful new wife anyway. I hoped she realized how dishy she was already.

Eloise Is Laying Eggs Again

Eloise, my pet cockatiel, is laying eggs again. She has done this at various times before, most often in the spring or fall. I always attributed it to the call of the season to which she responds like the wild birds that inhabit the nests scattered around my backyard. She does not have a mate so the eggs are never fertilized. No baby birds emerge from the beautiful oval products that she leaves on the cage floor. Still, like a good mommy bird, she sits on the eggs, fiercely protecting them from any disturbance, and eventually giving up on them when they don't hatch. Then I reach in and carefully remove the eggs. I feel bad for her loss each time.

My bird and I are about in the same place in our life spans. My egg production has stopped, though. No more monthly reminders of fertility. Eloise is doing this in reverse. As she ages, she is producing more than ever. It makes me wonder about the women who decide to have a family in their fifties. They have to go through so much trouble just to conceive. I think of the energy that is required to care for children. At twenty, it is a chore. At fifty, it is a different world. I wouldn't begrudge anyone having a child at any age but I can hear the conversation at preschool.

Twenty: "I think I'll go on the patch. It's easier remembering birth control once a week than every day."

Fifty: "I know what you mean. I have enough trouble remembering my Fosamax each Thursday but it is an improvement over popping the pill every day of the week."

And on the supermarket line.

Twenty: "I read that it is important to build strong bones early in life so I try to give my child leafy greens and calcium fortified drinks, and these chewable vitamins which she doesn't mind taking. I live in fear of scoliosis."

Fifty: "I can relate. I am chugging down that calcium orange juice like there's no tomorrow. My mother's back was so bent she got rich on the coins she found on the sidewalk. I make sure I go for a DEXA scan every year. Have you thought about getting one?"

Twenty: "Is that the bone scan? They don't suggest it before forty. I have a little way to go…"

And at work where childcare is an issue for every parent but the perspective may be quite different.

Twenty: "Thank goodness the day is almost over. I still have to pick up my child from daycare, make dinner, get him into the tub and read him his favorite book a dozen times before he unwinds enough to fall asleep. Then I can take a breath for myself."

Fifty: "Why don't you let the nanny take care of dinner and the bath? That's what she's there for."

Twenty: "Who can afford a nanny?"

At twenty I couldn't, now I can. Back then I felt that the most important thing I could do for my children was to be an at-home mom. But would the fifty-year-old me feel the call toward a different kind of fulfillment? Would a child's growth enhance or complicate life at this stage? Many grandmothers are forced into surrogate parenthood by circumstances and, while they love their grandchildren, wonder if they will ever have time for a personal relationship with themselves.

I sometimes wonder what Eloise would do if one of her eggs actually hatched. Would nature take over or would she take one look at the little featherless thing and say, I can't do this, like her birdie mother did after having one clutch of eggs after another, leaving the care and feeding to the human owners. Which is how we adopted Eloise. Maybe Mrs. Bird decided that she didn't have the energy to worry about breaking bones and nursing at the same time. I can understand that.

I believe that a woman has the right to choose the time for having a family, if she wants one at all. I'm glad, however, that I don't have to go through those particular conversations.

In a Word

This was a harsh week for the women in my family, starting with my being mistaken for my father's wife.

I was at the supermarket with my dad who, while he is still handsome and mobile and erect, has settled well into his eighties. He was just paying for his purchases at the checkout when the cashier turned to me and said, and I quote verbatim, "Is he your father or your other half?" She must have seen my jaw go slack because she quickly added, "You look so much like him. I know some women like to marry people who look like them." I informed her that he was my father and that I didn't think we really looked so much alike as I favored my mother. But the damage had been done. The rest of the day I kept peeking in the mirror for evidence that I looked thirty years older. Surely it must be glaring or she wouldn't have said what she did. Not that I wouldn't be happy to look that good in my eighties but I wasn't there yet.

"Ouch," my sister said after she stopped laughing. She tried to soothe my panicky feathers by telling me Dad doesn't look his age. He hardly looks over seventy, she assured me. The cashier probably thought I had married an older man. This did not make me feel better.

My sister didn't have long to console me, however, before she needed her own consoling. Later in the week, a man at my father's adult community thought my sister was a new resident. Technically she could have been, as she was past the fifty-five age requirement, but from the sampling of people we had been seeing, it was unlikely that anyone there was under seventy-five. I saw them talking. He was quite attentive. No one would have blamed me if I found this funny but my sister is only my senior by three-and-a-half years and that man, considering what I already experienced, might have been hitting on me instead of her. I told her that I bet he was just hoping that such a young chick had moved in.

Then there was the distress call from my daughter, who recently turned thirty-three and still looks young enough to be carded, because she had just been ma'amed. I remembered the electric shock that ran up my spine when someone called me ma'am for the first time. A layer of protection peels off like the skin of a reptile when that happens to a woman. She is left vulnerable to wrinkle sightings and the flash of a gray hair. She walks into a room differently, wondering who will notice the emerging ma'am in her. She feels the pulse of life's movement that she was unaware of until that moment. It will take a while for my daughter to toughen up again, to grow a new skin, but it won't be quite as tear-resistant as before.

"Service people are trained to call all women ma'am," I said. "It is respectful."

I don't know if that helped. As I said, it was a harsh week.

The problem is I'm not sure if it is respectful even if that is how the Queen and the First Lady are traditionally addressed. Is it showing esteem or is it just a label, a way of looking past a person?

I used to be amused when my daughter and I went out to restaurants because we always got exceptional service. The waiters never took their eyes off her even when I was ordering. I was the ma'am they didn't see. My daughter is too vibrant to be overlooked. She is not ready for labels.

I know the cashier was seeking a way to categorize us, to find an answer to her curiosity because my father and I weren't compatible with her expectations. She wanted to fit us into her worldview, to hang a tag on us that could be scanned and dismissed.

And my sister was probably someone's fantasy of the older, wiser, eternally virile man appealing to the younger, sensual woman. Just the age was shifted a little higher because our demographics have changed.

Labels, to sum up a person. A life in a word. One would think that the longer a person lived the harder it would be to find an appropriate label to express everything that had been learned and experienced. It seems to be the opposite. Aging creates one-liners. No wonder people hate to get older.

At the end of the week my husband and I went to our dance class and the first thing we heard was, "Oh, here are the good dancers."

Somehow I didn't mind this label at all. I stopped thinking about the supermarket cashier and her comment about my father. It was time to mambo. Whatever age I am, or look, no longer mattered. All I cared about was that rhythm. And movement. And the joy of dancing.

Another day I will ponder the inexplicable directions of life, which can't be expressed in a single word anyway.

Unless perhaps that word is "WOW."

Red Flight District

I painted my toenails red, a ripe, cherry red with a metallic shine. They are arresting in their brazenness. But only I can see them. They are nestled in thick socks on this cold winter day and hidden in duck boots as I shovel out from an unexpected two-foot snowfall. Still, I know they are there and the knowledge warms me.

This is not characteristic of me. I am not one for primping in general and rarely do I give myself a pedicure. If I polish my nails, it is my fingernails that get the attention; my feet get functional care. Yet, it has been a stressful year and it suddenly seemed important to do something different, to shift from taking charge to taking care. So I relaxed my feet in a gentle salt bath, scrubbed away the dryness on my heels with pumice and then lovingly applied the most outrageous color I could to my now pampered toes.

I find delight in my secret redness. It revs up my spirit and feeds my imagination. Red is a dangerous color, full of fire and possibility but most of all energy.

I am Circe and my red nails are my siren song. I will take advantage of any man unfortunate enough, or lucky enough, to come within my irresistible sexual aura. He won't have a chance.

Sometimes daily life needs a little flare. Too often I find myself operating on a pilot light, a warm body that keeps the coroner away but isn't what I would call living. There is just too much detail to attend to and not enough time for dreaming.

I look at my toes when I peel off my socks. They are still red, daring me to...what? I feel the thrill of them, these hot coals that don't burn. Maybe I have discovered something.

I am an inventor who has created a new source of heat, an energy source that will not deplete our earth's fossil fuels or cause us to rape the earth to dig it out. It is safe and non-polluting and abundant. It can be made on demand and simply applied. I will give this knowledge to the world for the greater good because to do anything else would be a crime against humanity.

I am taken aback each time I see its ten-toed intensity peeking through the white suds in the tub to surprise me with my audacity. I am enthralled with its brilliance flashing me to alertness, taking my thoughts away from the routine of my day. It is a hidden spotlight focusing on possibility.

I am about to go onstage. The audience is waiting, breathless. Each step I take brings me closer not to stardom but to expressing the message I have come to give. I can fade into the wings whenever I want to and shine whenever I choose. The audience bursts into applause at their first sight of me and as I begin, the hush is profound.

I know it's no big thing to have painted toenails, a whole industry is based on providing this service, but we each have our small pleasures that no one has to know about. These red flights of fancy help me connect with the wild part of myself that I keep so well under control. Does Clark Kent announce to the world that he is wearing a cape underneath his oxford shirt? Though I have to admit that I often, yes often, wondered how it fit so snugly under there. He knows who he is even if no one else does. He feels the power if the inner self to which others are oblivious.

I will not remove the polish. It will have to flake off of its own accord over the course of however long it takes. And chances are I won't replace it, at least not for a long time, because I don't want it to be so common that it fades into the ordinary. For a while I choose to feel the power of red without its heat and without its danger. I smile at this secret self and that smile carries me through the rest of the day.

Wait Training

I may have to avoid going to the supermarket for a while. I seem to be having issues with the cashiers. More than once I have found myself in a disgruntling interchange where I have been summed up and discounted.

The latest came after a day of speaking at an elementary school, when I ran in for some last minute groceries. As usual after an author visit, I was charged with energy, pumped with the excitement of showing kids how books are made and helping them create their own stories. I breezed into the store, scooped up what I needed, and went to check out.

I put the items I was carrying in my arms -- a half-gallon of juice, a pineapple, a head of romaine lettuce, a pound of tilapia fillet, half a pound of turkey breast from the deli counter, and a box of Quaker oatmeal -- on the belt. They weren't heavy, but they were wiggly so I was glad to put them down. The cashier looked at me as she was bagging my order and asked if the bag would be too heavy even though she saw that I had no basket and no cart. I told her no, it was fine. She cocked her head as though she didn't believe me and asked me if I was sure. Quite sure, I answered. I grabbed the bag and charged out the door.

It wasn't the kind concern of her first question that irked me but the disbelief of the second. She slipped from kindness into condescension. She was adding up her impression of me with the register tape: small equals frail, gray equals old. If I had a toddler on my hip or my hair had been brown instead of salt and pepper, she would never have asked.

I wanted to tell her, "Wait. Don't make such quick judgments about people because you may well be wrong."

I am probably stronger in my mid-fifties than I was in my twenties. I weight train and trek, which I never did then. My body mass index is in the athletic range. I go to a gym three times a week. Under the watchful eye of a trainer young enough to be my son who refuses to make any concessions at all to my age, I lift barbells and press more pounds than I weigh. He takes it as a compliment that my face is contorted and I am biting my towel. Pound for pound, he tells me, I am really strong. I trust his assessment because I can see the advancements I have made since I started at the gym. I know I am strong and I think my carriage and body tone reflect that strength. So I feel sideswiped by the casual assumptions of cashiers.

They are not the only ones who expect weakness from smallness. I have seen the look of disbelief on the faces of the other customers at the wild bird store when I head out the door unaided with a forty-pound sack of black oil sunflower seeds under my arm. And I once impressed a burly clerk in a department store when I hefted a box larger than I am onto my cart.

It's not that I aspire to be muscle-bound or unfeminine. I am quite willing to let a man hold open a door for me if he does it out of politeness, as I would hold it open for anyone behind me. I would be annoyed if he did it because he determined I wasn't able to open it myself. There may come a time when that is so but it isn't now.

I could probably dye my hair and avoid a lot of the assumptions that come my way. My mother-in-law did just that when her hair turned white at twenty-two. She knew how she would be perceived. There were too many important years of activity ahead of her before she would be ready to allow the judgments to be made.

And they would have been because we are a nation that likes to stereotype. We make assumptions all the time. We look at fat people and assume they are overeaters with no will power, not taking into consideration that perhaps there is a medical problem, an under-active thyroid perhaps, or that the person may be on prescribed steroids. We assume that all people want to be, would look better and be happier if they were thin. But we don't ask the people we are making assumptions about what their situation is or how they feel about themselves.

It used to be automatically assumed that women were bad drivers, certainly worse drivers than men. Some were, no doubt, but many were not. My mother drove assertively. She was always a better driver than my father, with a highly acute sense of direction. Everyone in the family respected her driving. And she was a patient and competent teacher when she taught me how to drive.

Older people are especially subjected to assumptions. Memory is often a problem as we age but it doesn't necessarily mean a vacant mind. And a wheelchair or a walker is not an accurate indication of mental acumen.

I know that cashiers and clerks and restaurant servers and all manner of service personnel receive training before they start their jobs. If I were in charge of those programs, besides the technical requirements of their positions, I would add one more category; I would see that they were proficient in wait training. I would encourage them to wait before they sum up a person, wait to see who a person is before they decide whom they see.

Getting Goopy

I have always had the tendency to be sentimental. Show me a kitten and I get goopy, reverting to preverbal cooing. Let someone tell me about a problem and I well up with emotion. I get choked up listening to toasts, tear at inspirational stories, and can be counted on to cry at weddings, baby namings, award dinners, gallery openings, and anniversary parties. This all before the unpredictable mood shifts of midlife. Now my goop quotient is even higher. When I watch the Olympics, each event has me sopping tissues. I cry for joy with the winner and weep in disappointment for the loser.

I can't venture into a card shop without breaking down at least once in the store. I can keep the whole greeting card industry in business by myself.

But it isn't just my natural goopiness that has been amped up since I went into menopause. My whole range of emotions has taken a quantum leap into expression. I find myself getting upset over the strangest things. The trivial and the profound are mixed together and one is as likely as the other to get me started.

My heart hurt the other day over a spaghetti sauce stain on my kitchen placemat. It seemed like just one thing too many to bear in this tough world of soldiers dying, impossible gas prices, and icecaps melting. Even as I recognized the ridiculous juxtaposition of topics, I still thought my heart might break unless I immediately removed the offending stain.

It is obvious that I am being hypersensitive, a condition that often causes me embarrassment. I know I am often helpful, nice most of the time, reasonably smart, and relatively cheerful, but let someone tell me that I am any of those things and tears cloud my eyes. I dissolved when a neighbor thanked me for helping her and told me I was kind. Gratitude washed over me. I felt as if the Pope had blessed me, and had to restrain myself from kissing my neighbor's hand.

Little comments that I might once have ignored or laughed about have me raging. I get incensed when anything is said about the laundry. My husband's request for clean socks can send me into a snit that could easily escalate into a major confrontation. He doesn't understand my sudden outbursts and looks at me as if I have lost my mind. Maybe I have. I certainly have been losing my temper.

I know this emotional irritability is part of the menopausal profile but it doesn't make it pleasant. It requires too much energy.

And yet...

I can see where there is value to this craziness. I think that the extremes allow women to ease up on the reins we bind ourselves with as our careers are developing, our children are growing, and our lives become intertwined with so many obligations. Menopause helps us give expression to the richness of emotion that lies within us. In the movie *Something's Gotta Give*, a midlife Diane Keaton's emotions were all over the place after she felt rejected by Jack

Nicholson's character. She laughed hysterically and cried just as vigorously. From that came some of her finest work both from her character and in her acting.

There is depth in our hearts that is waiting to be discovered. Anger expressed as rage is powerful. Love expressed as compassion is equally intense. Happiness expressed as joy is energizing.

I read that crones, the wise women we are growing into as we transition through midlife, welcome the sensitivity. It increases our ability to empathize. It helps us to embrace our wholeness.

That thought gives me breathing space within the turmoil. It also gives me the courage to do what a woman must do. Like brave the racks of greeting cards in a gift shop to look for that special birthday card for my friend. There were funny cards and serious ones, cards that made fun of aging and cards that reached for the spiritual. I chose two; the first card made me laugh out loud and the second was the goopiest one I could find. I cried all the way to the counter.

The clerk looked concerned as I rummaged through my purse in search of a tissue.

"Are you okay?" she asked.

I dabbed at my tears with the back of my hand because I had used up all my tissues while peering in the pet shop window at the poor little homeless puppies who were chasing each others' tails, and the kittens who were huddled in a sleeping ball.

"I'm fine," I answered with a shuddering sigh. "Just fine."

Wearing Crankypants

Warning! I am issuing an alert to my friends, to my family, to the neighbors, to the dry-cleaner, to the server who waits on me at lunchtime at the local deli, to the dog next door who is used to a friendly hello, to the person who gets lost on my street and might mistakenly think to ask me for directions and expect a coherent response; keep your distance. I am, as my kids say, wearing my crankypants today.

I am in no mood for putting up with obstacles, difficulties, or delays. I do not have tolerance for disagreements or differing opinions, nor have I patience for being helpful. This is not the day for the long telephone conversations I usually enjoy. There is no point in making a date to meet me because I will no doubt cancel it, which is probably just as well as I wouldn't be good company anyway. I am definitely in a mood, one of several that comes knocking at my door to drag me off to what I think of as the Midlife Amusement Park.

This park is not mine alone. It is visited by millions of menopausal women each day who, like me, are not particularly amused by its questionable attractions. No matter how many of us walk through the front gate, however, we experience the rides individually according to our hormone level and genetic makeup.

Here is a brief summary of what is in the park although I can only offer my own reaction to the rides.

There is the Nutritional Spin-around, the equivalent of the Tilt-a-Whirl ride that I used to love as a child but always made me so queasy I invariably threw up as soon as I got off. This version spins my nutritional needs in constantly changing patterns so that I end up taking enough supplements to occasionally make me want to hurl at the thought of another pill.

The Fifties Funhouse provides lots of frightening features, each of which is an entrance into the bizarre.

The Shifting Memory Walkway, for instance, the entry into the Funhouse, is distressingly unsteady to walk on. What starts out as a step forward can sometimes end up as two steps back. I am often tempted to turn around and go out the way I came in but with all the shifting going on, I can't remember where that is.

The Materialization Room is where unexpected things such as moles and hair pop up out of nowhere, which I find as creepy as the old vampires that leered out of the papier mache coffins of my youth.

And, of course, there is the Hall of Mirrors that can scare the pants off any woman. I scuttle back and forth from reflection to reflection looking for the one image that matches my perception of myself

The wildest ride of all, though, is the Climacteric, also known as the Hormonal Roller Coaster. It has twists and turns, heights that are exhilarating and low points that make a rainy day uplifting. It has never been my favorite ride, I admit. It throws off my equilibrium. While my teenage friends happily bought tickets to monster rides called Cyclone or Tornado, I used to go off to the fairway to toss Ping-Pong balls into fishbowls. They laughed at me but I didn't care. Not only wouldn't I buy a ticket for the roller coaster, but I wouldn't even accept one if it were offered for free. Now, ironically, I am on the biggest, twistiest, heart-thumping-est emotional coaster ride of my life.

Right now I am at the part of the ride that is climbing. It is annoyingly slow and frankly, it is getting on my nerves. Yet as exasperating as the climb into irritability is, it is actually an improvement over yesterday's mood when I walked around wearing gray-colored glasses seeing the clouds in silver linings. Every penny I found on the street was tails up and I seemed to focus on the spent flowers and not the opening buds. Knowing that depression is common during menopause is little comfort at the bottom of the ride. At least when I am grouchy I am actively engaged in life, interacting with it, grappling with it in my climb back up the track.

I am certainly not easy to be around, however. I gave the letter carrier a hard time about delivering so much third-class mail, mostly sweepstakes come-ons, even though I understand my clogged mailbox isn't his fault.

"Doesn't it bother you, having to carry so much junk?" I griped.

He shrugged his shoulders. "It's job security," he said.

I had the bank teller recount my withdrawal because I wanted fives instead of twenties and although I had a good reason, I wasn't about to explain why.

I cut my sister off mid-conversation because I wanted to change the subject and politeness became a casualty of my mood.

This grumpy state will eventually transition into a high point where, at the top of the coaster, I will be able to see and appreciate the larger view and perhaps take some of that joy with me as I swoop down again through the sentimental and melancholy phases of the ride.

I know it is coming and I look forward to it. I will welcome it with wine and laughter. I will call my friends and smile my way through the day. I will catch raindrops in my hand and pretend they are diamonds.

But for today, watch out world.

I'm wearing my crankypants.

Night Prowling

It is three-thirty in the morning according to the glow on the clock radio. The outside world is dark and silent, still too early, though not by much, for the birds to start their morning concert. It's not too early for me, though, to be prowling the house as I often have lately, searching for the one spot that is cool enough to relieve the night sweats or sufficiently comforting to lull me back into sleep for a few hours before it is time to begin my day.

I shuffle down the hall toward my daughter's former bedroom. Sometimes changing where I lay my head helps me calm my inner turmoil. I stretch out on the bedspread, tuck my toes under an open-weave afghan, and wrap my arms around a fresh pillow. It is soothing for the moment, until I cook the pillowcase with my internal oven and with a disgusted grunt, toss the pillow across the bed. The stuffed lion that guards the room stares at me with its yellow cat eyes. I can't tell if it is disapproving of my mini-tantrum or is sympathetic behind its imperturbable expression.

"Is it too much to ask for one good night's sleep?" I growl to the lion. It keeps looking at me, unblinking, a fluffy Sphinx.

I try to meditate but I am too out of sorts to focus. My mind jumps from one idea to another. I begin my yogic breathing practice. It quiets me down until another flash works its way up through my body and leaves me dripping again. I am desperate for sleep.

I sigh as I watch the sky lighten. It will be a tired day, one of many I have experienced in the last few years. I think of the Statue of Liberty, holding up her lamp day and night, never sleeping. No wonder the first words on her base say, "Give me your tired..." She knows about fatigue.

I give up trying to sleep. I go into the early morning stillness of the kitchen and make myself a cup of herbal tea, which I take upstairs and set beside the bathtub. Then I fill the tub with soothing bubbles and a few drops of valerian, settle myself into the welcoming water and imagine that I am floating on a calm tropical sea. The scent of the tea wafts over to me. I reach for the mug and slowly sip.

Fully awake now, but more relaxed, I relish the warmth of the bath and the pre-dawn hours. Once I am over the annoyance of not sleeping, I actually like having the time to contemplate. My thoughts expand and I let them flow freely. They settle into a peaceful place where I can appreciate the gifts of this age.

It has taken a while but I finally can see the positive changes that are taking place. The hot flashes I rail against are burning away my fears. They remind me of the power that resides within. I am more outspoken than I was, less shy about interacting with my world.

The sleepless nights force me to rest during the day instead of darting around like a jackrabbit through the desert brush.

My moods, ah my moods, how human they make me feel. Yes, I am edgier than I used to be but I am also more alive. Being outrageous makes me laugh and laughter brings joy.

My prowling is over for today. I dry myself in the soft folds of a voluminous bath sheet, then lovingly apply my favorite vanilla-scented lotion. I snuggle into the blue terry robe with its worn elbows. The desperation is gone as I tiptoe downstairs again, savoring a few last solitary minutes.

Peeking out my kitchen window, I greet the birds who are now gustily chirping up the sun. The daddy cardinal is at the bird feeder as usual, a bright beginning to any day. My sweet cockatiel, Eloise, has just come out of her cage and is preening her feathers in preparation for breakfast.

I feel the house stir itself awake. There are mouths to feed. The laundry is calling. My work is drawing me, suggesting stories and bringing me characters as I hustle through the morning routine, eager to get to my computer.

"Good morning," I say as I pass the wide-eyed lion on my way to my office. My feline guardian is comforting in its unwavering presence.

It is the beginning of another grand day.

Reflections

Finding Perspective

I am off to meet my friend for lunch. She and I have the good fortune to share a birth date. Each year we celebrate with a birthday luncheon to commemorate another year's events and another year of friendship. We started our tradition when we were in our thirties. It is hard to believe that was over twenty years ago, that more than two decades have zipped by.

We don't need to refer to age. We know the numbers. She is a year older; I am a year younger. My friend tells people who inquire, because that is the first question they tend to ask when they hear it is your birthday, that she is now fiftyish, more ish than fifty, and that's about right. Whatever our age, we never feel it.

We give each other presents on this day. This year I am giving my friend a copy of a book I'm reading and feeling excited about. I know if I like it, she will, too. Whatever she gives me will be something I will love, though I always think of our meeting as the best present of all. No matter where we go, what we eat, what we exchange, it is the conversation, our connection that is the celebration.

I have noticed that as time passes, our conversations are drifting into new territory. Our lunchtime chats have moved on from discussing the difficulties of raising a family to a reporting of how our children are doing in their independent lives. We talk about our careers less often than about the supplements we are taking for hot flashes, arthritis, and cholesterol. To glucosamine or not to glucosamine, that is the question, and an imperative one when achy joints are asserting their claim to attention.

What we discuss most, though, is the shifting understanding at this time of our lives. At each turn of a year, the usual becomes new based on added awareness and the new becomes expected because change is a daily occurrence. We are discovering what is really important, assessing where we are going, and making alterations in our circumstances and our attitudes. It is not always easy. What served us in our pre-menopausal years is not always helpful now. We are living lives we never could have envisioned in our younger days.

One thing we both find enchanting is how alive we feel. Despite the physical matters that occasionally demand our focus, the forties and now the fifties are wonderful decades full of power and capability and confidence.

But the best part is a new perspective. Wrinkles, shminkles. A lot of living went into producing them. So what if our bellies won't disappear? We have had babies, for crying out loud (and they did), beautiful children who have grown to be incredible, creative adults. Surely that is a fair exchange for such a grand result. And if we need a nap now and again, well lots of people take naps. Most European countries have a tradition of an afternoon respite and Europeans are considered chic.

I love getting together with my birth mate, but all of my fiftyish friends are delightful. We are all at different stages of cronehood so we can mentor each other with the wisdom of having been through each phase. In sharing our lives and support, we gain the courage to examine the choices we have made in the past and move forward with the options we have for the future.

I am not concerned with any of that today. I am only anticipating how glad I am to have friends who are loving and fun to be with as we all go on this journey. I will toast my friend with iced tea and wish her a healthy year, a year filled with things that make her smile and keep her growing, as I know she will wish for me. Then we will get down to the good stuff – the details of the year that we have both just moved out of and our excitement for the year we are moving into. It will be a wonderful fiftyish birthday.

Stretching With the Seniors

Once a week I volunteer in an assisted-living residence to do stretching with the seniors. They show up faithfully, eight to twelve of them depending on their current state of health. They come to class pushing walkers, leaning on canes, hobbling on swollen legs. But they come. They come to work out kinks in arthritic shoulders and get circulation back into aching muscles. They come to help their limbs move again because their joints have stiffened over the course of the week.

They are bundled in shawls and sweaters even though the space we use is warm. Once we start, though, reaching out with our arms and stretching our legs, turning our torsos and breathing, breathing, their circulation revs up and the sweaters come off. Pale cheeks show a rosy tint and furrowed brows begin to soften. They do as much as they can. Some days are better than others but they are here.

"Em's asleep," someone whispers.

She has fallen asleep mid-rotation, her leg extended and her toe pointed.

"That's okay," I say. "She'll catch up with us in a minute or so."

I am used to the sleepers. Two or three regularly take catnaps in the middle of our session. I don't wake them. I know that most of my group has trouble sleeping through the night. Although we meet at 11:00 in the morning, some have already been up for six hours and are ready for a break.

Often they complain about having muscles spasms in their calves that keep them awake. I tell them that it sometimes happens to me, too.

"But you're so young!" they say.

Compared to them, I am. We just celebrated one woman's ninetieth birthday. She is the average. The residents' ages range from the high seventies to the low hundreds. My fifty-six seems young but we are all part of life's continuum and I get muscle cramps like the rest of them. We talk about taking calcium to prevent the spasms and how to press acupressure points when a spasm hits. We massage our muscles, warming them up so we can use them in the rest of our workout.

"Today we are going to dance," I tell them as I put the CD I brought into the player. The room fills with swing music and some jazz and blues.

"We not only get to dance but we have free entertainment," one woman says.

She means me. The music has me bopping around the room as I do in my kitchen whenever I put on music. I encourage them to do the same, to keep moving as much as they can through the day so that they won't stiffen up so much. Pain keeps them immobile and immobility feeds the pain. I help them to stretch in time to the music, to move every part of their bodies. One man, who can barely move his shoulders, is shrugging in half-time. The grimace on his face soon turns into a smile. Others move slowly in their chairs, some to the beat, some randomly, but it doesn't matter as long as they are moving. One of my regulars who broke her hip and is now using a walker says that the stretching helps her as much as physical therapy.

Em stirs from her catnap and is surprised to hear the music.

"We're dancing, Em," I say.

Her eyes brighten.

"We used to love to dance when I was on the farm," Em says. "Even the horses and pigs danced."

"The pigs, Em?" someone asks.

"Especially the pigs," she says. "Did I ever tell you about my pet pig?"

She did but we listen anyway as she shakes off the remaining sleepiness, reaches out in time to the music and tells us about her dancing pet pig. We love to hear Em's farm stories. They always make us laugh. Our inner beings need exercising as much as our bodies.

I have Steve Martin's happy feet and happy everything else. These people, with their aches and complaints, their challenges and struggles, add to my day's happiness. They give me faith in the strength of the spirit despite the body's limitations. They stretch me as much as I stretch them.

Rabbit Lessons

Shortly before six, I go into my kitchen to prepare dinner. We eat fairly much the same time each night. Our bodies are attuned to being hungry on a schedule. As I wash my hands at the kitchen sink, I glance out the window to see if the usual passel of squirrels is scavenging and to check if the finches are feeding. Our dinnertime seems to be their time to deplete the black oil sunflower seeds we provide for them, an expense my husband complains about but doesn't really seem to mind. Maybe I'll be surprised by the yellow-shafted flicker I saw only once but for which I have been on the lookout ever since. Or perhaps the red-winged blackbird will make an unscheduled appearance.

As soon as I look outside, I know that dinner will be late. Today there are rabbits. Two of them, no three. Three beautiful rabbits at the base of the bird feeders chowing down on the crumbled end of a loaf of bread I had moments ago scattered. It must be a family, I think: two parents and a teenager.

Of all the creatures that inhabit my backyard, I am most fond of rabbits. Over the years I have learned a lot from them. They have taught me about the value of being still and listening to what is going on around you rather than running about blindly before you assess a situation. They have shown me the beauty in just being yourself. And they have helped me to understand about the commonality of life. Pretty heady stuff for such tiny professors.

One of the adult rabbits leans over to nuzzle the younger one. Is it the mama? I know some human men who would do that with their children though more often it is the mother who is the open nurturer. My son would disagree. He is an unabashed nurturer as are two of my nephews. If they were present, we would all be crowded at my sink peeking out the kitchen window, dying from cute. But I don't know about rabbit relations. I suspect that wild nature has more structured interactions.

I turn away from the outside scene and begin gathering ingredients for dinner for the people in the house but make the mistake of looking back out the window. Another rabbit, another teen, has joined the group. The organic, red-leaf lettuce I am holding would taste just fine to the outside family and I am willing to share but I don't want to scare them off by opening the back door. I'll save some to put out the next night. Besides, they seem to be enjoying exactly what they are eating.

Once again, I am about to turn away and get on with the business of cooking when a fifth rabbit hops up to the feast. This one is a baby, smaller than the squirrels milling around impatiently waiting for the lapins to leave. It could fit in the palm of my hand. I watch its tiny mouth try to engulf one of the larger crumbs. The bread is too big and keeps dropping. The rabbit keeps trying. I am rooting for it.

"Go little rabbit," I say through the glass between us, encouraging it the way I would my own child who was attempting a difficult task. "You can do it."

The rabbit swivels its ears toward the sound. I don't think it can hear me but maybe it can sense my positive intentions for it. It finally succeeds in biting off an edge. It tucks its cotton ball of a tail underneath and sits contentedly chewing. I am contented, too, watching this exquisite little expression of Mother Nature.

But now I absolutely must prepare dinner. I hurriedly reach for the skillet. I was going to make a more elaborate meal than this will be, accompanied by a salad of mixed greens and baby spinach and homemade applesauce for dessert, but I have spent so much time rapt in rabbit suppertime, the human dinner will have to reflect a simpler plan. A mélange of thinly sliced cheese, medallions of zucchini and sautéed rice in a delicate tomato and wine sauce enhanced with pine nuts and roasted red peppers. In reality, it is a meal-in-a-pan. I feel a little guilty at the menu comedown.

My husband notices the time on the clock when he comes in. I point to the window. He looks out and nods then unfolds the newspaper and starts to read.

"Ahh, slop," he says when I finally place the revised creation before him. "My favorite."

I laugh and I kiss him on the forehead. It echoes Mr./Ms. Rabbit's affection for their rabbit child. I don't know what prompted that demonstration but I know what triggers mine. I feel a welling up of love for this man in my life who understands about rabbits without my having to tell him.

I sneak a last peek out the window before sitting down to my own plate. Having eaten their fill, the rabbits are scampering across the yard, back to wherever their haven is. I silently thank them for their presence and the lesson in appreciation as I happily dig in to this perfect, though different and somewhat late, dinner.

Beachcombing

Well, another weekend was spent not buying that beach house I always say I want.

I am surrounded by friends who have taken the plunge. They all love it. They tell me how they enjoy long, lazy days on the sand. They tell me how sweet the air smells when the wind blows in from the ocean and they rhapsodize about the endless hours they occupy beachcombing. There is nothing like it, they assure me.

So my accommodating husband, and I, once every couple of years, go out and look at houses. We almost bought a large, five-bedroom Victorian in a small shore town last time we house-hunted. It had everything I wanted: many bedrooms, a wraparound porch, closeness to the beach. I could already feel my toes wiggling in the cold Atlantic. But the weekend before we were to commit to it, neither of us slept. The few times we were able to drift off, we would suddenly awaken in a cold sweat.

I understood that taking on another house was a big responsibility. It meant assuming another mortgage and doubling up on the furniture. We would be hosts to drop-in guests when we wanted privacy, an inevitable consequence of shore ownership, said our friends, but not unpleasant. Is that what was holding us back?

We examined our motives but didn't feel that any of that was sufficient to keep us from buying that second home. What was it then? Maybe we should do it anyway. I knew that my husband would have put aside any misgivings if I said I really wanted the house. After the second sleepless night, however, I looked at my husband and then let my dream house go. My feelings bounced from relief to grief and back again.

We took a vacation later that year. It wasn't to the shore. We went to Africa on safari. We had two glorious weeks of being pampered and of connecting with nature in its wild state. It was only two weeks. We traded year-round beachcombing for this? we asked ourselves. Yes, we did. Had we bought the property, we probably would have stayed home and bought furnishings for the new house. It would have been fun but we would not have watched cheetahs on the hill stalking a lone impala. Or drank champagne ten feet away from lounging lions. There would have been no elephant charging us in our backyard either, and no incredible African sunsets.

The next year we went to Peru and walked in the footsteps of the Incas in Machu Picchu. There was no ocean to swim in on that trip but there was a llama to follow on the narrow trail that snaked along the side of the magnificent Andes.

This year we went to Malaysian Borneo. I danced with the Iban, the native headhunters, swam in rivers and bathed under a waterfall. We visited with baby orangutans and saw a mother turtle lay her eggs.

We love traveling and can't imagine a year without a trip to a place that takes us out of our culture or time or language.

But it crept up on me again, the longing for the shore. So we ventured back into the real estate market. We discovered that the house we almost bought was now worth at least twice what we would have paid for it. The market had changed since our last foray into it. Did we regret it? Maybe a little. We looked at listings and checked out neighborhoods.

Once again, at the possibility of buying a house, we turned to each other with that unanswered question in our eyes.

My thoughts drifted off to the places we had seen and those we had yet to see. There would only be those two weeks and, if we were lucky, another week somewhere in between. We would have our photos and our memories and the new friends we made but it wouldn't be the consistent, comforting presence of a place at the shore.

Is having that comfort what I wanted at this time in my life? Was it what my husband needed? Was it wiser to buy our shore house now since the world has become less safe and traveling so uncertain? We both knew. This would not be the year for the house. We would choose our destinations differently but we would go.

I still love the shore and one day, sometime when the greater world isn't so insistent, perhaps we will settle into a sandy place of our own. Until then, my definition of beach combing will have to be broadened to exploring more than the coast at our fingertips. Different times in our lives call for different responses. Now that our children are grown and while we are able, travel is our comfort and our joy.

When the travel brochures come in the mail, I look them over eagerly. My husband says, "Where do you want to go?"

I gather the catalogues together. I will take my time reading them before I answer. They hold treasures inside like the shells that encase the tiny sea creatures that wash up on the sand. For now, these are my beaches. I can't wait to start combing.

Facing Fear

I was telling my friend about planning my latest trip, to the Galapagos Islands, aboard a hundred-foot yacht. I also told her about how I have this tendency toward getting seasick.

"Do you notice a pattern here?" she asked.

"What pattern?" I said.

She reminded me that when I went to Machu Picchu, I ended up hugging the side of the mountain half scared out of my mind because I am prone to height freight. And that although I complained often and loudly about how I couldn't stand the hot flashes I was experiencing, I chose to go to Borneo which, in case I had forgotten, was on the equator and about 180 degrees in the shade.

"I repeat," she insisted, "a pattern."

"Hmmm," I said.

Not a profound response but a thoughtful one. Have I been purposefully doing those things that I most fear? Not long ago I went hot air ballooning knowing that the only way for the balloon to go was up. Up high. I thought I could scrunch down in the basket beneath the balloon but it was a lot shorter than I envisioned and too crowded for me to sit on the bottom. I imagined falling out and breaking bones

I couldn't even pronounce, if I survived at all. It turned out to be pretty tame and incredibly beautiful but until the balloon was aloft and we were floating calmly above the treetops, I was a wreck.

So why did I go? At this time of my life when I could be avoiding my fears so successfully, I seem to be rushing headlong into them. My friend was right. I went ballooning quite specifically because I was scared.

Some people do risky things for the adrenalin kick. That isn't my motive. Growing up as a shy child, I spent so many years being afraid of so many things that I figure it's about time I started working through them. That doesn't mean I intend to go downhill skiing or bungee jumping any time soon. I have enough stuff to work around without giving myself a guaranteed heart attack.

I am not the only one doing this. Another friend went parasailing. Her fear was not being up in the air but coming down. What if the boat towing her didn't stop and she was dragged in the water like a fish trying to get off a hook? Would she get hurt? But she went anyway. I told her next time we would go together so she could calm me down when we went up and I could buoy her up when we came down.

I'm learning that the physical fears are easier to deal with than the emotional ones. Saying I'm sorry for the insensitive things I may have said or done to a dear friend is not easy. Forgiving someone for hurting me and truly letting the hurt go is a toughie. Speaking up for myself is perhaps highest on the list of fears. I don't like dissension. But there are times when it is important not only to stand in your truth but to express it as well.

I am learning to speak up to my father, to tell him the things he needs to know without being hurtful. I can tell him when he is wrong about something, which I hadn't been able to do until recently, and to encourage him to do things differently. Sometimes it works, sometimes not, but I speak up all the same.

When I am asked my opinion, I give it. Why not? Maybe I'll be disagreed with, but that is part of the give and take of conversations and makes them more interesting. I don't have to worry about being right all the time.

And I have come to know that I don't need to be perfect. Or the best. Participation is more satisfying than perfection. Chances are that there will be someone better than I am at almost everything. Especially when I am learning a new skill. Whatever made me think I had to know how to do something perfectly from the very start? It kept me from doing lots of things. But no more.

Fear has become an amber caution light to me rather than a red stop light. I look around and if there isn't an authentic reason to be afraid but only my own reluctance, I may go for it. The best pattern for life may just be no pattern but a willingness to be in the world whatever comes.

Maybe that is what I have been doing without realizing it. And discovering a new, exciting world in the process.

Stringbean Sisters

Mid-way between the cantaloupes and the red peppers in the produce section of my local market, my attention was caught by a mountainous display of stringbeans. I hadn't planned on buying stringbeans but that mountain drew me to it.

There was one other woman at the stringbeans. She, like me, had her hands in the mountain of pods, but our picking styles were different. She was delicately selecting one or two beans at a time. I dove in, grabbing up handsful and then discarding those I didn't want. We were after the same thing, though. Not the longest but the best beans, with the right amount of moisture. I could tell by her pursed lips that she did not approve of my approach. Maybe she thought I was after her beans but I wasn't. In fact, I tried to keep over to one side. Bean picking can get territorial. By the tightness on her face, I suspected she could use a friendly word.

"Am I in your way?" I said. "I'll move over."

"No, no, you're fine," she said and gave me a half-smile. She seemed to relax a little but continued to protect her private space.

Another woman came and carved out her own picking area. She was tall and had the advantage of being able to reach the higher, virgin beans. She would pluck one from the pile, inspect it visually, put it in her plastic vegetable bag. Then she would pluck another. A very deliberate style.

Two more women showed up and set to on the middle of the pile with a focused intensity. One of them hummed quietly as she picked. When they caught me looking at them, I smiled. They smiled back.

Now there were five of us, all picking companionably beside each other. It reminded me of the Sesame Street song that went, "Oh, there are five people in my family…" For some reason, I felt connected to these stringbean women. They were my picking sisters and as quirky as the members of my real family.

When the tall woman caused a cascade of beans she said, "Avalanche!"

We laughed, all except the reserved woman who seemed like she wanted to but couldn't allow herself to join in the spontaneous interaction of strangers. I could understand her hesitation. When I was younger, I never would have had the nerve to speak to strangers like this, to enjoy the instant camaraderie that sprang up between us. On this day, that shyness seemed silly.

"Quite a mountain," I said to no one in particular.

"Yes," agreed the hummer and then added, "Isn't it a beautiful day?"

"Are you having company?" I asked when I saw her beginning to fill a second bag.

"Oh, no. This is for my kids. I'd rather have them eat stringbeans than candy."

That led to a general discussion on healthy foods versus fast foods and a brief exchange of recipes among us.

The other mid-mountain woman told us that she was having a family dinner. Sixteen people. She had invited her cousins and an older aunt and uncle from over in Pennsylvania.

"I thought after the horrible attack in New York it was important to have my family all together. Why wait for a special occasion?"

"You're right," said the tall woman. "The world is too uncertain to take family for granted."

We started telling the stories we had heard about rescues and near misses. Then we went on to talk about our children. The first woman seemed more and more uncomfortable with the casual conversation that had arisen. She tied her bag and moved off toward the apples. I shifted my position for a better selection. I was glad to have the extra room but it felt as if the circle were incomplete. One of us was missing.

It was odd that no other people approached us as we talked and picked and laughed. Didn't anyone else need string-beans? There must have been an energy that enclosed us in this friendly exclusion. We might have known each other for years by the ease with which we spoke.

Wouldn't it be nice if this could be the normal way of meeting people, I thought. I knew nothing about these women and they knew nothing about me but it didn't matter.

I picked more beans than I really wanted because I was reluctant to let go of the unexpected camaraderie.

The first woman, whom I noticed hadn't moved more than a few feet away, came quietly back to the mountain. "I think I'll get a few more," she said. She held up her almost full bag almost apologetically. "Just a few," she muttered.

"There's plenty left," I said.

I moved over again, to make a place for her. The others adjusted their spaces too, welcoming back the prodigal sister. She looked at us gratefully then took the place we made for her at the stand and in the conversation.

I don't know how much time had passed but when the produce clerk came with some more boxes to replenish the supply of stringbeans, we simultaneously backed away, tied up our bags, and put them in our carts. We had taken all we needed, of beans and of support. We wished each other a good day and went down other aisles. The new batch was for another group, another meeting of other sisters who would find the strings of connection in a mountain of beans.

Long Distance Daughter

The telephone rang and I knew with a mother's instinct that it was my daughter calling. Her home is not so far away, only about three hours, a relatively easy visiting distance. But it also is not around the corner, not convenient for getting together for lunch or afternoon tea. So we chat on the phone.

Today we shared memories of a family cabin up in New England where each summer we spent time with her grandparents. We talked about picking fresh vegetables for our dinner from the garden her grandmother so carefully tended. She remembered the wooden footbridge from where she and her younger brother threw crabapples upstream and then watched to see which would come out first on the other side.

We reminisced about the steep, rocky slope that led to the real log house waiting in welcome at the top of the hill and the trips to Glendale Falls where we walked on the slippery rocks while the water striders skimmed past our legs, and where we once met a group of burly campers bathing in water so cold we could hardly bare to stand in it. There was great fondness in the memories for both of us. We often find comfort in these periodic dips into remembrances.

Sometimes we discuss the world's problems and come up with our own solutions for world peace. Not today. Today our personal worlds needed some attention.

We talked about the term paper she was researching for a graduate class she didn't really want to take but needed, and how hard it was to spare the time to gather the material, no less write the paper. I griped about the manuscript that came back in the mail after an incredible eighteen months. We commiserated about the swiftness of our days, hers spent in teaching, mine in writing.

But there was comfort in this, too, knowing that no matter how large a pity party we threw for ourselves, the person on the other end of the phone line would not think any less of us.

It wasn't always this way, this easy communication, between us. When she was a junior in high school, we started a quiet war. Nothing she did pleased me and everything I did embarrassed her. When she left for college, it was to our mutual relief. I have heard this from many mothers, that their relationships with their daughters was so frayed by the time high school graduation came around, everyone was glad for the separation.

Then their daughters would come home after their first semester away as different people. Happy to be back. More loving. More understanding. Distance softened the strain. Teenage adversaries turned into women friends through the alchemy of perspective.

When I speak with this woman, my daughter, now, I am careful with her feelings. I treat her with the respect I show any of my contemporary women friends. Part of this shift comes from knowing that should I cross the line back into controlling parent, she will have no qualms about letting me know it is inappropriate. But the greater part comes from the genuine pleasure I get from this new relationship. Slowly, I am releasing the roles I have played in her life to become a spontaneous, joyful companion. I still provide emotional support when necessary but it is the verbal kind and I find that I am freer to ask for my daughter's advice, her compassion, her wisdom in a woman-to-woman way. Age is no longer relevant – it is understanding and experience that counts. We have much to teach each other and even more to share.

I know this long distance daughter will not be coming back to live near me. Her life has taken her in other directions. The telephone keeps us connected.

Our conversations, once or twice a week, are long. We never plan them to be, it just happens as one topic segues into another. There are points when it is possible to end, to let the tenuous electrical impulse go, and we recognize the moments but we let them slip into a few minutes more, reluctant to say good-bye quite yet.

When we hang up at last, we each sigh and are glad that we live in times where it is possible for long distance daughters and mothers to give each other long distance hugs. Our teatimes will remain fantasies that stretch over the cellular and digital miles, at least for the foreseeable future. In our busy lives, however, those three hours that might have been an insurmountable barrier to our maintaining such a relationship have been bridged by the telephone. Our knowledge of each other as relatives, as friends, and as women grows.

And so does our love.

Wedding Dress for Sale

Some years ago, when it looked as if my daughter were in a serious relationship leading to marriage, a beautiful wedding dress came up for sale at an incredible price. It was a designer gown customized with lace and beads by a professional seamstress for her own daughter. I encouraged my daughter to try it on. Even though the dress would need some alterations, I could see the potential, and my eyes misted looking at her in it. She wasn't sure about the dress, but in my mother zeal I bought it for her, had it dry-cleaned, and put it away for the event that seemed imminent.

Then that relationship ended. The dress stayed packed in its vacuum wrapped state. I put it in the storage closet in the basement. It remained there unthought of for a couple of years until another relationship stirred up my memory of the billowy dress waiting for its chance to shine. But this was not the right relationship and the dress remained in its airtight packing.

When my son became engaged, my future daughter-in-law wanted to try on the dress. We unwrapped it from its tissue-paper nest. We fluffed it up and spread out its layers of satin and lace and sequins. It had been tucked away for so long, I had forgotten what it looked like. It wasn't the dress for her. It was too much of everything -- too much material, too much design, too much not her. So we folded it again and arranged it carefully back in its box.

In the meantime, I realized that the dress was too much for my daughter as well, mostly too much emotional baggage. No matter how much we might try to alter it, there would always be the memories of past relationships shimmering in the sequins and former expectations trailing behind with the train. I should have waited. My love was too controlling. It hadn't recognized that my daughter had truly grown up.

A wedding dress is more than the material it's made from. My own wedding dress was not glittery at all. It was a sheath with embroidered silk leaves that ran down the front in three simple rows. I can't pass it on to my daughter because it wasn't preserved and besides, would she want to get married in her mother's gown? Looking back at the photos in my album, the dress is lovely but does not feel like the right one for my daughter even if it were available.

One woman I know said she borrowed hers because she couldn't see spending so much money for one evening. She never regretted the decision but happily paid for a new gown when her daughter got married. Another woman got married in a plain white suit at city hall and had a simple but exuberant house party with her friends afterwards instead of catering an extravaganza. And still a different bride wore a comfortable cotton caftan with a string of flowers crowning her hair, the better to play volleyball unencumbered at her wedding picnic.

It is more important for a bride to choose her own dress, be it fancy or plain, high fashion or casual, than to have it chosen for her even if it comes with a mother's loving intentions. A wedding dress, after all, is the bride's personal expression of celebration.

So I am looking for someone who would love to own a perfectly beautiful traditional wedding dress, worn only once. The price is exceptionally low but too high for my daughter to pay. She will find her own dress when the time comes. And whatever it costs, it will be exactly the right amount.

Home Retreat

I had never been on a formal retreat, off to some special location where peace and silence envelop you from the moment you step inside. I know others who have and they tell me about the healing that takes place within that atmosphere. So this weekend, my friend and I decided to experience one. It wasn't at a holy place. It didn't cost spa prices. And we didn't have to sit in traffic to get there. We merely carried a tray bearing a Victorian teapot filled with English Toffee herbal tea and a couple of cups and saucers up to the small room I call my office and closed the door.

When we lived near each other and had the luxury of constant contact we would often come together for reading, sewing, cooking, enjoying the company of the other as the work was done. Just our mutual presence was calming. We would fit in our many discussions between classes at the college we both attended or up and down the grocery aisles as we did our weekly shopping.

We live in different states now. The miles that separate us are a physical ache that we feel despite the telephone calls and frequent e-mails. We make plans for several trips a year back and forth as couples (our husbands are friends, too) but this time, we needed more than a social visit. So we closed the door and took this mini-retreat away from chores and husbands and the outside world.

We have been friends since we were teenagers. We met at the Pioneers, a newly formed summer day camp program that promoted service and taught us fundamental skills in working on the land. As campers, we leaned how to plan a project, measure, saw, hammer, plane, and use a posthole digger. We learned teamwork and how to see a project through to completion despite complications such as an attack of angry bees when we accidentally knocked down their hive, and having to transport ourselves and our equipment onto the site when there was no road.

But we learned even more basic skills. We discovered how to gauge a person's trustworthiness and how to be someone who could be trusted. We stretched our physical limits to uncover a new competence and channeled our intense teen energy into something positive.

After eight weeks of hard work, we had helped to complete a sturdy amphitheater for outdoor plays, skits and meetings that would serve the campers of future summers, which it has. By then we had also forged a friendship that continues more than forty years later, a friendship that is stronger than we would ever have dreamed it could be.

The hours that passed in my office brought us back to our camping years and earlier as we dug into the soil of our childhoods. I had insight into her issues and she was able, competently and lovingly as always, to shed light on mine.

We had talked about these particular subjects other times, so it surprised us that they resurfaced. Perhaps it was the events of 2001 that created the climate for our own insecurities, the terrorism of the present echoing the terror of the child. I think it was more that we were unearthing the deeper shards that had been lying hidden in old emotional ground. We were comfortable with these archeological digs of the psyche and excavations of the soul because of the trust we had developed over the years.

As evening approached and we sipped the last of our tea, we knew hadn't solved the world's problems but we were able to look at our own through new perspectives. We found solace in each other's words as we had as teens. The intimacy we shared was a fond recreation of the old discussions we used to have and loved so much, a re-treat for us both.

And I finally understood the call to go on a retreat. For a short while, the small room in my house, my tiny office with its scattered papers and unread magazines, was transformed into a holy place for us, a place of sanctuary and comfort, of gratitude and love. It became a place to contact that deeper connection that comes when the world is quietly set aside and the sharing heart is the loudest sound heard.

Kitchen Dancing

I love to dance. I'll put on a CD and move. Classical or klezmer. Island drums or swing. It doesn't matter. Music moves me in more ways than one. The kitchen floor is my stage, the ceramic tile providing a smooth surface for graceful glissades and a sturdy one for the pounding I give it choreographing my own Broadway numbers.

Over the years, I could sometimes coax my husband onto this impromptu dance floor for a slow dance but we have learned from experience, beginning with our wedding, that we don't dance well together. We seem to have an abundance of left feet, which usually end up on one or the other's toes.

All that is changing. I signed us up for dance classes. He agrees to go only because our son is getting married soon and we will have to dance, at least once, in front of almost two hundred of our closest friends and relatives. I don't care what reason gets him there. We are dancing.

My husband complains that it is impossible to count the beats, do the variations and feel the music at the same time.

"That's multitasking," I tell him.

Women are used to it. Folding the laundry and helping with homework. Cooking dinner and talking on the phone. It comes naturally.

"I'm a focused kind of guy," he says. "I do one thing at a time."

"Good," I say. "Do one thing. Dance."

We learn the steps in class but we practice at home. In the kitchen. The room really isn't big enough for an elegant foxtrot and it does put a crimp in an enthusiastic swing but it will do.

It was difficult at first. Between my jittery energy and his resistance, our individual needs frequently clashed. I would resort to leading when he wasn't forceful enough, which irritated both of us. But we understand now that we each have our parts. He leads. I do the flourishes. With practice we are learning to sense each other's strengths and respond to each other's timing. Our posture is getting more confident. We have stopped staring at our feet, willing them to go where they are supposed to instead of being surprised by where they might end up.

I am grateful for the impetus to learn together. I have been feeling deprived all these years, relegated at formal affairs to marking out steps against the back wall, but was not able to impress my husband with the need to dance. His body remained still in his chair while mine was moving, squirming, aching to be up there in the middle of the energy. No more. I intend to dance from now on. The wedding is the excuse but the reason is that something inside me at this time in my life says I must move.

I tell myself that because I sit writing at my computer for so much of the day, my body needs a release. It sounds logical, though I know my need has nothing to do with logic. It is an inner pulsing that calls for movement.

I think this passion for dance is partly rooted in childhood. A desire long delayed. When I was a teen, I wanted to take ballet lessons. My mother wouldn't let me. She said I was too skinny, too frail, to dance. So as my friends took the bus to their class, I practiced the lindy in my basement with a friend down the street. We danced to our forty-fives and then rewarded ourselves by polishing off a Sara Lee chocolate swirl poundcake.

But the teenage years are long over. What I see now is a population growing older and becoming more sedentary. In an assisted living facility where my parents lived, I saw how many ways people could stop moving. Sometimes inaction was physically based: a stroke depriving muscles of movement, a damaged heart causing every exertion to be painful, brittle bones making any action dangerous. Yet lack of movement was often caused by lack of interest or fear of trying something new. Rigidity of thought expressing itself in rigidity of body. I found myself starved for movement after a visit.

My husband puts on a Benny Goodman CD. Who better to swing to? We work our way across the tile and laugh our way through our mistakes. We make up combinations that we are too shy to do in front of our instructors. At least until we perfect the timing.

I love the grin on my husband's face when we finish a pattern and come out on the right step. Even better, the panic has begun to ease when we come together. I can see where it might actually be pleasurable one day to be a dancing couple instead of a couple of dancing bears.

And dancing has drawn us closer, even after thirty-seven years of marriage. There is a lot more hugging, more innuendo, more delight. Maybe it's just our endorphins running wild. Dancing is, after all, an aerobic exercise that releases those wonderful chemicals of euphoria.

But I see it in a different way. I think of it as freedom. Freedom from the seriousness of daily existence. Freedom for the exuberance of life. It is a guiltless pleasure that reminds me of the joy there is to be had in simple things. Simple things like dancing in the kitchen.

Mom's Jewelry

When I was a little girl, I used to look through my mother's jewelry box. There were treasures hidden inside. Whenever my parents went out for the night, I would spread out Mom's jewelry on their double bed in order of preference, starting on the pillow and working my way down the bedspread. A rhinestone studded pin in the shape of a crown. Slithery golden chains to wrap around my arms so I could pretend to be Cleopatra. More rings than I had fingers. There were earrings that dangled halfway down my neck and those with tiny pearls I could clip on my ears and feel like an elegant lady. At that time, the most elegant lady I could think of was my mother.

What I loved best of all, though, was a bracelet with milky stones that my mother called moonstones. If I were lucky and my mother wore something else that night, I could have the bracelet for myself until I went to bed. I would hold it up to the window to compare it to the moon. The moon was always bigger but the stones were brighter. They seemed to glow more brilliant as the moon got larger until, at full moon, they were so beautiful, I thought they must surely be worth a fortune. One day when I was grown up, I decided, I would wear the moon on my wrist, too, and be an elegant lady.

When my mother died, the bracelet became mine. I sent it to a jeweler to be polished and thought that it would become one of my treasured possessions, a part of my mother that would shimmer with my childhood memories. It came back with the same lustrous glow I remembered. I looked at each perfect stone linked in its place along the old-fashioned silver setting. All these years later and it was still beautiful.

But I couldn't wear it. It was now tied up not with my mother's elegance but with her disappearance. Her physical body survived into her seventies but Alzheimer's disease claimed her personality and spirit. There was no elegance in the slow passage into dementia, in the anger of her despair. There was nothing elegant about having my mother, the woman who had so carefully tended to her hair and her nails, looking like a vagrant and smelling worse than a sewer. I could not separate the two images. The little girl was too devastated and the adult too traumatized to be comforted by the moon.

I put the bracelet into a plastic bag with some of my mother's other jewelry, none of which I would wear, and stashed it in my closet.

It was there where my grown daughter found it one day when she was visiting.

"Ooh," she said. "When did you get this?"

"It was Grandma's."

She held up the bracelet and let the light shine through the translucent stones. She turned the stones around to peek through them the way I had all those years before. As I watched her, I saw them again through my child's eyes. I remembered my mother in her glamorous days with her dark hair and wide smile getting dressed for an evening out. I saw her again as she turned toward me and held out her arm.

"Can you help me?" my mother had asked.

I reached out to fasten the clasp on the moonstone bracelet, which glamorously circled her wrist, and was rewarded with a hug when it clicked into place. I could still smell the perfume that lingered on my fingers after my mother left, a heady aroma that I associated with the secrets of grown-up life.

I snapped back to the present when my daughter asked, "Can you help me, Mom?"

Once again, I fastened the bracelet only now it was around my daughter's delicate wrist. It looked perfect on her, elegant the way it was supposed to look.

My daughter and I found the necklace that matched and scavenged through the other pieces of my mother's jewelry, taking out whatever attracted her. We cleaned them and packed them for her to take home. Now and then I will see her wearing something from Mom's jewelry box and I am glad.

Maybe one day I'll be able to wear my mother's jewelry again though my Cleopatra days are gone. I will look for my own elegance as a woman grown and tested, as a mother passing on life skills to her children, as a person discovering her value as the decades unfold. I will remember not my mother's craziness but how she tried so hard not to be crazy. And when I turn toward the moon, I will know that no matter how beautifully a jewel glows, it is the human spirit that truly shines.

Grand Pig, Cat, and Kids

As my daughter's biological clock ticks, so does mine. She is a mother wannabe, I am a grandma-in-waiting. I never thought I would be in this position, yearning for a grandchild. In fact, I wasn't even sure that I would want a grandchild to be brought into this iffy world. But nature has other priorities, I guess, and now that I can no longer have a child, I feel the pull of an infant as yet unknown.

At the moment, though, my daughter is focusing on her career even though she has these longings. I am confident in her understanding of her own timetable for having children. Kids deserve to have parents who are ready for the commitment it takes. I applaud her responsibility. I am proud of her principles.

So I lavish maternal attention in other directions for the moment.

I give my daughter's dappled guinea pig extra green beans when he comes to visit and make sure I have the kale he loves to eat. When the weather is nice, I take him out for a pig-nic in the backyard where he munches the grass with intense concentration. Every now and then he stops chewing to check on me, making sure that his protector in this wide world is still within scooting distance. I gently rub his velvety ears. His babbling-brook sounds of contentment remind me of my daughter's sweet baby gurglings. I pick him up carefully and hold him against my chest. Like a swaddled infant, my grandpig works up a mighty heat that warms me through my shirt and melts my heart. He is the best guinea pig in the whole world.

My son is getting married, but I have no expectation of a grandchild there any time soon. So I jabber to his orange tabby, cooing to the cat as if he were a baby. This grandcat of mine looks at me with caution. He is not used to such endearments from my son. He is cared for and loved and occasionally called "Baby" but rarely goo-gooed at.

I never used baby talk with my own children, so this is an unexpected development. I remember scolding my parents when they produced the same kind of nonsense talk to my son, telling them that he needed to hear real language so that he would learn to imitate proper speech. They looked at me as if I had gone temporarily demented. Babies are meant to be babied, they said. I stood firm. They shook their heads but complied. What would they think of me now if they heard how I spoke to my grandcat? But I wasn't in grandma mode then and didn't understand how more than speech comes through a well-intentioned coo.

I am not obsessing about this. Most of the time I am not even thinking about it. Yet there are times that I can feel a space inside me that could very nicely be filled with a grandchild. The feeling arises most during weddings and family gatherings when my aunt is sure to ask, "So when?" It is an all-purpose question that covers most of life's progression. "So when -- are the kids going to get married, are they going to have children, are you going to be a grandma?" And should there be one grandchild, it is the question that will be asked about any further grandchildren. The comment underlying the question is that I'm not getting any younger. I know that. Who is? Maybe that is part of my yearning.

But my aunt isn't the only one baby-prompting. The feeling sometimes is present at the mall where pint-sized shoppers with bigger than wide eyes greet me as I go from store to store. It is amazing how cute babies are. Any babies. People babies, puppies, kittens, baby rabbits, ooh they are soo sweet. What pwecious widdle feets they all have.

Yes, well.

I can hear my parents laughing.

I look at this as valuable practice time. I am learning how to make my house grand pig, cat, and kid proof. It is all pretty much the same. What shouldn't go into one tiny mouth really shouldn't go into any. The tail that can sweep a loved Lladro off a table could just as easily be an exploring hand. I even have a baby gate to keep the cat, and any possible children who might stray into this house, out of trouble.

I say none of this to my daughter or my son. They live in a world filled with choices. Perhaps they will choose not to have children at all. That will be fine with me. No pressure. I just want them to be happy. My daughter is responsible for her own clock as I am for mine.

But when she is ready, I will be, too.

Swimming With Turtles

I have this strange connection with turtles. It started when I was four years old. I had a turtle named Myrtle. She was a plain, Woolworth's variety, one of a pile of turtles the store crowded into an aquarium in its pet section. There was nothing to distinguish her except that she was mine.

One day my sister and I took Myrtle out of the bowl to play with her, and somehow Myrtle vanished. There was no way she could have avoided being spotted on our white kitchen linoleum, but she simply disappeared. It was as if she had cast a spell and became invisible. We looked all over but could not find her.

For days we walked around the apartment with our heads down, partly because we were sad but mostly so that we wouldn't step on her should she decide to show herself. We finally accepted that she must have been sick and crawled off to die somewhere. Two weeks later, when we were eating dinner, she scuttled out from behind a kitchen table leg. It was a mystery to us how she had kept herself alive with no food or water. But there she was, good old Myrtle, brassy and bold.

I met my next turtle fifteen years later. I was driving to the supermarket when I saw a rock crossing the road in front of my car. The rock was actually a large box turtle that must have been displaced by a housing development. I stopped in the middle of the street to block another car from running it over and took it home. I kept it in my bathtub, feeding it raw ground beef and lots of greens, until I learned that it was illegal to harbor a box turtle in my state. I released it in a wooded area near a pond and wished it a good life.

Surely that was the end of my turtle connection.

Yet, ten years after my last turtle encounter, I was on my way to pick up my son at his pre-school when another rock stepped out onto my path. Another box turtle! I brought it to school where it had an extended month-long visit with my son's class. Then it was let go on the teacher's farmstead.

Why had two big, beautiful box turtles crossed my path when most people never come face-to-face with a turtle of any sort? Could my turtle encounters have been coincidences, chance meetings without further significance or did they mean something?

Being a firm believer that everything has meaning, I looked up turtle lore and found that turtles have always been seen as mystical creatures. They are a symbol of longevity and they bring good luck into a house. Some say that if you dream of a turtle, it foretells of an incident that will bring amusement or an improvement in business. Long life seemed like a good idea and good luck was always welcome. I thought it would probably be wise to pay attention the next time a turtle popped up in my life.

As soon as I started looking for them, the turtles stopped coming. I thought perhaps we are only allotted so many turtles in a lifetime. They seemed to have done the job, though. I couldn't tell about the length of my existence but my life had been blessed with good fortune in many ways.

The turtles hadn't finished with me yet, however. I was swimming in the warm, luxurious sea during a vacation in Hawaii when I felt someone beside me. I looked up expecting to find another swimmer and there was a sea turtle not three feet away. I held my breath, afraid that it would disappear. It was a huge creature more at home in the water than I was and graceful in a way that made my best sidestrokes look like wild flailings. We looked into each other's eyes and continued to swim, side-by-side, for another five minutes. Then the turtle dived. I followed but it quickly vanished along the sandy bottom. I propelled myself out of the water and sprinted across the beach to where my husband was reading, oblivious to the incredible adventure I just had.

"I am changing my name!" I yelled as I ran. "Call me Woman Who Swims with Turtles!"

I told him the story but I could not convey the sense of privilege I felt. Our mutual swim was a companionable bonding, a sea-earth connection that made me feel that I belonged to the turtles, to their 175-million-year existence on this planet. I was expanded in a way that left all boundaries between living creatures behind.

The experience brought to mind Myrtle and every turtle I had met since. It took me a while to connect the turtles with my life but when I finally did, I realized that they were all there at significant points in my life: shortly before my family moved, on the eve of my first major trip abroad, when I sent my son off to preschool. And now, a magnificent being was affirming my spiritual journey.

Maybe there will there be more turtles at my life's junctures, maybe not. If one presents itself, I will thank the turtle as is only proper, and keep my eyes open because something will change, no doubt for the good.

And I must believe in the mystical nature of the connection for why else would my messenger of change come in the form of something that has remained the same for eons?

Smiled Into Morning

In the early morning of our thirty-eighth anniversary, long before the alarm clock crowed its greeting, I lay awake wondering. How is it possible that we have kept our marriage happily going for so long when half of all marriages end in divorce and most of those never see a decade?

We don't do the romantic Hollywood things. We don't kiss good-bye when one of us leaves and there is usually no welcoming kiss upon return.

Since neither of us is a morning person, our first words spoken at the beginning of each day tend to be mere grunts of acknowledgment of the other's presence.

We don't usually celebrate birthdays with presents or parties. I might get an anniversary card or not and I might or might not give one. Probably a passing hug will be the only recognition of the event.

My mother's advice when I was newly married was never to go to bed angry. Do not let an argument linger overnight, she said. It would only be worse in the morning. Yet there were many nights that I wanted nothing to do with my husband and I am sure he often felt the same about me. On some occasions, the distance between us on our queen-sized bed was not nearly enough as I huddled on the mattress edge. I would think of my mother's words, too mad to heed them.

But there were other times, when we would sit together reading companionably, that a peace would steal over me and I would think how wonderful it was to have the space to go into our own thoughts and still be so sweetly connected.

There are daily hugs, not contingent on a holiday or reason, that make me melt into this man who has long been in my life.

All this floats across my awareness in the new light of dawn.

Still, I wonder where the fulcrum is, the balance point that keeps everything stable. Could it be quantified? Does one hug balance out two grunts? Does the excitement of a trip to Paris neutralize the tedium of making oatmeal every morning?

I turn toward my husband on this anniversary day, my thoughts still heavy with unanswered questions. He reaches for me as he comes out of sleep. His eyes slowly open and there, in the first contact of the day, he smiles.

And now I know what keeps this marriage finely balanced.

Despite the tips into anger and the dips into quietude, the bumps of anxiety and the tumults of passion, there is a fulcrum of delight at being with each other, of knowing and accepting the other person even when not agreeing. Of recognizing this other person as an integral part of a beautiful life.

It is a balance that allows for looking lovingly once again into the face of my husband of thirty-eight years and being smiled into morning.

Wake-Up Call

The phone rang at three-twenty a.m. It is a rare call that brings good news at three o'clock in the morning. My mind immediately went into high mother gear. Did something happen to one of the kids? My sister and I often talked about how we never wanted to get a dreaded early morning call and here it was. I croaked, "Hello?" into the receiver, hoping it was a crank call and I could just hang up and go back to sleep.

No child was in danger but the news was horrific anyway. My sister's house was burning. She and my brother-in-law were standing out on the sidewalk in front of their home in their bathrobes watching smoke billow through the roof above the master bedroom where minutes ago they had been asleep in their bed. He had grabbed the cell phone on his way out while my sister rounded up the dog and cat. The fire trucks were on the way. My husband and I threw on our clothes and rushed over. We had no idea how we could help but we had to be there anyway.

By the time we arrived, the street was lined with ladders, hoses, helmets, and men. My brother-in-law was walking around dazed, in bedroom slippers a neighbor had given him; he hadn't stopped to look for shoes. Their best friends, who live a couple of blocks over, provided jackets and gloves and warm companionship in the chilly pre-dawn.

There are no words to describe the emotions that run through you as you watch your house burn down. My sister tried.

"All the pictures are gone," she said.

Those few words carried a world of meaning for me. When our parents broke up their home in the north to move to Florida, we found a carton of family photographs put out for the trash. We had rescued a century's worth of photos and divided them up, reliving our family's history as we looked through them. There were fading images of immigrant relatives who braved the ocean to start life in a new land and photos of favorite family members who had died over the years. There were pictures of our children at all different ages that flooded us with memories and often made us laugh. We gave our cousins the photographs that we knew they would want and felt relieved that we had spotted that carton before it ended up in some anonymous landfill. Now that was exactly where they would go, charred and singed and crumbling into ash.

My sister had lovingly framed family portraits on her bedroom wall, albums on the bookshelves, photos in the drawers. There were no walls anymore, no shelves, no drawers.

The paintings she and her husband had collected over forty years were destroyed. The jewelry she had chosen so carefully was under tons of rubble as the first and second stories tumbled two floors down into the basement.

In the space of the few minutes it took them to get out of their house, they had lost their past. Two more minutes inside, the fire marshal told them, they would have been overcome with smoke and lost their lives as well.

Each time it seemed as if the fire were over, more smoke would pour out of some other part of the house. The sound of shattering glass brought our attention to a new plume of black smoke escaping from the guest bedroom. The firemen aimed the hose and tore at the eaves with hooks. We couldn't take our eyes from the scene. It was compelling, in a strange way, like pressing a bruise to see if it still hurts. We know it will but we do it anyway.

We didn't notice when the sun rose and we didn't feel its warmth. We were shivering, from the cold, from the distress, from our horror at what was happening, and the fear of what might have been. We let the firemen continue their work and turned our backs on the smoldering shell to warm up in their friends' house.

My sister focused on the fact that all the living beings survived and not on the idea that she no longer had any possessions. While many people offered her temporary sanctuary, it didn't alter the fact that she was, in actuality, homeless.

She had a rough day when the house was due to be razed. The frame was too unstable and dangerous to remain standing. What was left of the floors hung unsupported and dangled oddly over the yawning chasm below. She understood the necessity for it but didn't want to see the final demolition. We went out to lunch instead, sharing salads and gratitude and making plans for the next house. It will take at least a year before she will have a place of her own again. She and her husband are rebuilding on the same lot because their neighbors were so caring they don't want to leave the area.

She laughs when she makes reference to something she has, or rather had, and that happens often because she is a generous person, always lending clothes and pots and books and jewelry. The inclination is there but not the objects. She knows that they will come again, in time. What is more important, she sees who and what are valuable in her life.

One of the things she has come to value is life's irony. It was one of those dreaded three o'clock phone calls, not their fire alarm, that saved their lives. Their phone system had a feature that caused their phone to ring when the electrical system failed. When it rang that morning at just three o'clock, waking them, my sister went into the same mother alert I had, thinking the worst had happened to one of her children. When she saw the smoke and knew that the house was on fire, she did not think of what was about to be lost; she thanked the powers that be that her children were safe.

"The fire put everything in perspective," she said.

That phone call gave them the gift of those two life-saving minutes. It gave me the gift of a safe sister and brother-in-law. And it opened all of our eyes to the incredibly delicate balance between being alive and just living.

Making Peace with My Name

My father asked me today if my name was a burden to me.

It used to be.

Anyone given an unusual name when I grew up would understand.

I was born into a world of Susans and Carols. People never pronounced my name right and I was too shy for most of my childhood to correct them. I lived with being called Frieda, my cousin's name, or answered to mispronunciations that made me cringe. The one time in junior high school that I worked up the courage to politely tell my teacher how my name was actually pronounced, she withered me with her icy glare and said that in her day, a pupil would have been so grateful that the teacher knew who she was that she wouldn't care how her the teacher said her name. She continued pronouncing it the way she pleased and I was too cowed to say another word about it.

I also got teased a lot by the kids. One boy asked if my name was a flower or a state. Another said it sounded like a disease.

Girls were sometimes kinder. Either they made the effort to find out how to say my name or they ignored me completely, which was fine with me. I just wanted to get lost in the crowd.

I used to envy my girlfriends who had names that didn't sound as if they were spitting when they said them. Norma. Ellen. Brenda. I bet they didn't cry in their pillows the night before the new school year started, anticipating the agonies of being introduced to a whole new group of teachers and kids.

One year, my best friend decided to change her perfectly good and pronounceable first name. She asked everyone to call her by her middle name, Candace. Then she shortened it to Candy. What I wouldn't have given to not only possess a middle name but to have one I could shorten! As I struggled with my given name, I wondered, Why in the world would my parents give me such a name?

Actually, I knew. My parents named me for my grandmother. They gave me the most beautiful name they could think of. But in Susan's America, I was doomed.

Somewhere along the way, there was a shift in naming. Children born in the nineteen-sixties often had names like Summer or River. I fantasized about what life might have been like with a name like Spring. I daydreamed that I was called January or even better, the French Janvier. Ooh, that coated my tongue like melted chocolate. So what if I was born in July.

Asian names started cropping up in my neighborhood. And beautiful Hindu names. African-American names that sang. And all kinds of spellings for even the most common names. Jennifer was spelled Gennifer or Jennipher. And no one cared!

Over the years, my sensitivity to my name eased. I stopped feeling the knot in my stomach whenever introductions were made. I thought it might even be an advantage to a writer to have an unusual name. No one could pronounce it, but they sure never forgot it.

Then one day, my whole perspective changed. I had the privilege of being invited to a Sufi wedding. The bride graciously introduced me to the imam who had performed the ceremony. When he heard my name, he gasped. Then he reached out for my shoulders, pulled me gently toward him, and kissed me on both cheeks. He said that the syllables of my name mean Heavenly Paradise. Wow. Who could ask for a better name?

My name is still pronounced wrong most of the time and people still make funny comments about it occasionally but it doesn't seem to matter any more. In fact, now that I no longer try to or even want to blend into the background, I rather enjoy the attention I get. I have made peace with my name.

All this ran through my mind in the second or two after my father asked his question. Should I lay my name experiences before him? Would it in any way help that shy little girl who no longer existed? I knew what I would answer.

"No, Dad, not any more." I said.

And of all the stories I might have told him, I chose to retell the one about the Sufi wedding.

Backyard Observations

My backyard is a wildlife sanctuary. I once counted twenty-three different varieties of bird visitors. There are squirrels, of course, and rabbits, chipmunks, an occasional raccoon or skunk, a more than occasional neighborhood cat, even a stray groundhog. We all coexist in a small suburban yard not far from a busy main road. I am the largest being in the grouping but my size doesn't seem to frighten anyone. I've often pondered this lack of fear. Is it possible that they sense, in some kind of nonverbal communication, something about me that says I am harmless?

When I work in my garden, the birds fly off to a nearby bush to wait for me to finish so they can return to their continual eating. If I take too long with the weeding, they start to chatter, scolding me for my inconsideration. As soon as I leave, they are back feeding. One feeder looks like an apartment house for purple finches. Sparrows, goldfinches, chickadees, and the fly-in—fly-out juncos prefer the other feeder. The ground beneath is littered with broken husks and tossed-out seed, most welcome by the ground feeding doves, grackles, redwing blackbirds, and the hairy beasts.

The rabbits tolerate me. They sit on the lawn placidly munching clover. They don't bother to keep me in view. They turn their rounded backs toward me as if I posed no threat to them at all, which is absolutely true although I don't understand how they know this. Once a baby rabbit came close enough to sniff the big toe sticking out of my sandal. "Boy, are *you* going to get a scolding from your mother when you get home," I said to it softly. No fear. Only when I moved my foot slightly did it scoot away.

Even the calico cat who shows up on a regular basis from somewhere up the street knows it has nothing to fear from me and saunters past my window quite without concern.

That cat and I once had a head-to-head confrontation. It was bedeviling a chipmunk that was trying to hide behind the trunk of a skinny swamp maple and was yelling its heart out in terror. I shooed the cat over the neighbor's fence but it came back. I shooed it again and waited. The cat found a hole in the wood and stared through it at me with perfect patience. As soon as I looked away it returned, so I kept eye contact. We spent an hour in this standoff until the chipmunk worked up enough courage to break for its hole. But the cat comes back, not at all discouraged from the hunt. It looks curiously into my window to see if I am home and inclined to bother it that day.

My rescue didn't give me any points for power, however. The chipmunks scurry from their summer home in the herbs to their winter home in the woodpile. I might as well not be there as they hurry, hurry, back and forth, their cheeks puffed out with seeds. If I am relaxing on the concrete patio, they run right past me, sometimes hopping over my feet, through the pachysandra, behind the arborvitae, and they disappear into the ground.

I tell myself it means something that animals take me for granted. It feels important. I am glad that my yard invites rabbits even though I rarely have produce for my table. Besides, rabbits teach me many things.

There was the time I left my snack, a dish of dry, whole grain cereal on the patio while I went to water my newly planted black-eyed Susans, and came back to find a baby rabbit helping itself right from the dish. I let it eat its fill and then distributed the rest to the birds. I would have worried had the dish been filled with junk food. It reminded me that I am responsible for the food I eat, to keep it wholesome enough for a rabbit and other wild guests to enjoy.

Rabbits have taught me about companionship. When I get too close, they scoot away. Yet, the day I was down in the grass plucking clover from the lawn by hand, a rabbit came nearby to graze. We were no more than three feet apart. As I moved slowly from spot to spot, the rabbit shifted with me. We were just two beings grazing in silent, though amiable, company.

There is nothing that needs to be done here. The trees grow by themselves--or they don't. The flowers bloom with or without my care although they thrive on gentle attention. But don't we all? The animals come and go as they please, chase each other in turf battles, teach their young to survive.

I have spent the greater part of five decades thinking that I must be in control of all aspects of my life. Yet this backyard doesn't need my input. I garden for my own pleasure, and share the environment with its natural inhabitants who are perfectly capable on their own. It is calming to observe how everything works even without my effort. In this high-energy world, sometimes observation is all that is required.

Letting Go of the Key

I am walking around the house on the eve of my son's wedding. This is a happy time. He is marrying a woman I love, who I can see loves my son. I know they will be happy together and I am enthusiastically looking forward to this celebration. Yet nostalgia has overtaken me.

Each room holds his energy though he hasn't lived home for quite some time. There are reminders everywhere of his presence, of his growing up, of his connection in the family.

I remember holding my son moments after he was born. He worked so hard at lifting his head to see me. We looked into each other's eyes and I was captured. I knew I would love him forever. It was as if he had given me the key to a golden city, his care and well being transferred to my hands. I accepted the key with gratitude and anxiety. Would I be able to fulfill the trust presented to me?

I see pictures in my mind of the three-year-old being pulled around in a wagon by his sister and her friend while he sits serenely snacking on a baked potato. I feel his tiny hand in mine as we walk down the street. He needed me then for the basics of life and

I felt fortunate to be able to provide them. But the key was only on loan and I knew it.

I replay his first day at preschool when he wanted me to stay. I knew I was handing him back his key, temporarily. He was leaving me, reluctantly at first but eagerly soon after, and taking his first steps toward independence. Each day when he returned, the key was transferred back and we both felt a little easier.

I see him biking down the street on his first two-wheeler, his abundant brown hair blowing in the wind and independence shining on his face. I watch him going off to school with his friends with hardly a backward glance, and I remember how proud I was of him. He was growing up, as he was meant to.

Over the years he chose to keep his key more often, returning it less. But there was always that invisible thread that made us both keepers of the key. When trouble stuck, that thread thickened and we shared the responsibility the key demanded. There was no one to blame when he fell off the climbing gym at nine and broke his wrist. Risking is an important part of life's experience. For a while, though, as I made sure he received the proper medical care and comforted him when he hurt, I held the key. As soon as his wrist healed, he was back in possession and back climbing.

When he was diagnosed with diabetes after a bout with the flu at sixteen, no matter how I wanted to protect him and spare him from the disease, he was the one who had to care for himself. He took over his daily shots and monitored his blood sugar. I tried to hold onto the key by planning his meals and keeping on top of his monitoring but he wouldn't let me. He had too much living to do and was often gone: on weekend camping trips with his scout troop, on school trips, overnight at his friends. He knew that he was in charge so I backed off.

As I wander in and out of rooms, his bedroom still loaded with his boyhood furniture, the toy room stocked with his favorite games, the den where he often fell asleep while watching television, I question my motivation. I have been only a peripheral part of his life since his college years really but still I felt that bond that was evident at the beginning of his life. Am I trying to hold onto him? I wonder. Am I being the cartoon mother-in-law?

My friend said that she felt the same nostalgia when her son married. It wasn't anything against his fiancée I was feeling but a shift of allegiance. Now he will be consulting his wife on the major questions of life. He will present me with his choices and not his quandaries. His father and I will no longer be his next of kin and his birth family will be less important to him than his newly formed family.

I am glad. I've seen the results when a man was not able to make that shift. His children always felt second best and his wife came up short in any comparison. It does not make for a secure family. What that man didn't realize was that his first family was the background for his chosen family. They would always love him. He didn't need to keep earning their love. He was just never able to claim his own key.

My nostalgia tour is over. I mentally wrap the thread around the jewelry box that holds the rings for tomorrow's ceremony, the rings my son had entrusted to me to hold until his wedding day. I do it carefully and deliberately so it will not tangle. My love for them both makes letting go of the key not a reluctant duty but a sacred rite of motherhood.

Looking Through New Eyes

My father always says I have an overactive imagination but I couldn't have imagined what was about to happen that bright winter morning as I drove him to get a haircut. It was the beginning of a day of errands we were planning to do together. We were simply chatting when he asked me, "What's wrong?"

As far as I knew nothing was wrong, only I kept reaching up to brush something away from my right eye. It was probably just a hair passing across my face but I couldn't seem to find it to get rid of it. I probably needed to get a haircut, too.

Suddenly, a shadowy haze washed over my eye. Then thousands of tiny black dots burst into my field of vision, fogging my focus. I caught my breath. What just happened? I wondered. I had never experienced anything like that. It wasn't painful but it certainly was distressing. I pulled into the barber's parking lot and let Dad go in while I waited outside to assess the situation.

The dots settled down a little and seemed to spread out while a shadow washed over everything, eventually gathering itself into a form. It looked to me like a giant squid had taken over my eye, it's body lodging in the upper right and its tentacles spreading wildly to the left. I couldn't rub it away or move it. Each time I shifted my gaze, the squid's large body swam into view. This is just a floater, I assured myself. I have had floaters in my eye before. But this was extreme. And I was now getting lightning flashes at the edge of my vision. It was like a storm at sea only this sea was my eye.

When my father came out, I told him that our day together would have to be postponed. I drove him home and then went home myself. Surely whatever was going on in my eye would clear up in a short while. It didn't. This was something that needed attention.

Three hours later I was in the ophthalmologist's office diagnosed with a condition common in eighty and ninety-year-olds.

"How is this possible?" I asked. "I'm only in my fifties."

"It also seems to happen in very nearsighted people," he said.

I have been nearsighted all my life. I faked needing glasses by squinting my way through kindergarten. Everyone made fun of the kids who wore glasses and I didn't want to be one of them. I memorized the eye chart in first and second grades when they tested our vision in class. My trick worked until third grade when I wasn't able to get an advance look at the chart. I tried bluffing my way through it, guessing that the top letter was the usual large E. Only this time the test was not to identify the letters because every letter was an E, but to tell what direction the Es were facing. I had no way of knowing as I could barely see the printing on the chart. I was fitted with my first pair of glasses that very week.

It took many years of teasing before I felt at ease with my eyes, comfortable to the point where my nearsightedness was just another aspect of who I was. I came to appreciate my ability to see even though it was diminished from other people's vision. At least I had sight. Now and then I would stop and realize how much I actually could see within the blur.

Now I wasn't so sure I would have the privilege of sight in both my eyes.

I had a condition known as posterior vitreous detachment with vitreous hemorrhage. Part of the transparent gel, the vitreous humor, that fills the eye had liquefied and was floating around my eye. The retina in back of the eye registers light. The material that had broken free was floating around and blocking light from hitting the retina forming shadows, my squid. These floaters, as they detached, tugged at the connection with the retina, causing the lightning flashes. The black dots were the result of a blood vessel breaking when material detached.

I learned that the condition was permanent but the dots and floaters would settle down a bit in time and that most people learned to look around them. For the next six months, however, there was an increased risk of retinal tearing or retinal detachment. The ophthalmologist sent me to see a retinal specialist.

The retinal specialist confirmed my condition and added that it was important to watch for uncontrolled light flashes, which could signal retinal tearing. Should I see a gray curtain move across my eye, I was to come in immediately. That would indicate retinal detachment, which if untreated, could lead to loss of vision.

The first few days I walked around with a patch over my eye because it was easier being one-eyed than squid-eyed. I started asking myself how I would adjust to only having one eye. I tested my depth perception. I paid attention to how I processed color and assessed how I did with a variety reading materials, including my computer where I wrote and earned my living. I had to prepare myself for being blind in one eye, just in case.

When I told a couple of friends about what happened, I discovered that they had the same thing. One was diagnosed five years ago, the other ten. I never knew. They assured me that I would be able to see reasonably well again. At least within my normal parameters.

In follow-up appointments, the dots receded and the floaters, while still there, had taken on different, less obtrusive forms. They began to look like they were in a free-for-all mitosis, the process of cell division I remembered from biology class. Less obtrusive but still a lot of activity. Then they settled into a couple of small jellyfish that followed the movements of my eye. Annoying, perhaps, but I am often able to ignore them. Fortunately, there was no retinal tearing.

So I can see again, not the same but adequately. I have to admit, though, that I was shaken from my complacency. While I cannot remember a time when my sight was good unaided, I took my eyes for granted. Yes, they needed help but they worked and I really didn't think much about them. Now I do.

I am looking at my sight through new eyes. With gratitude. With concern. And with an added measure of respect.

Despite what my father says, my imagination is not good enough to imagine the rest of my life without the use of my eyes.

Forgetting and Remembering

As soon as my shiatsu practitioner pressed into the acupressure points along my spine, my body remembered what I had forgotten. Last year I had promised myself to get a massage on a regular basis, at least quarterly. But without a scheduled appointment, a year had passed since my last one and now each pressure point was a testimony to my forgetfulness.

My memory has become somewhat erratic. My friend says that it isn't memory loss due to aging, rather that our brains are so full there isn't room to hold anything more. If something new comes in, it pushes something else out.

Perhaps. It is something I would want to believe because it is preferable to the alternative of losing my little gray cells. But didn't I hear (I forget just where) that we use only ten percent of our brain capacity? If I used up all the cells devoted to remembering appointments, why didn't cells from the other ninety percent of my brain do the decent thing and volunteer? There is no point in memory cells being tied up in quadratic equations that I never use when they could occupy themselves more productively by calling up the title of a good movie I want to recommend or reminding me to send birthday cards out on time.

I don't want to hear about right brain, left brain. It's all *my* brain and I should be able to direct it to function according to my needs. If my left brain wants to do math, let it remember how to divide three-quarters of a cup of flour by one third so that I can alter a recipe accurately. Or calculate the amount of time it will take me to get home when I'm stuck in traffic and hungry.

I don't want my right brain feeling smug here. I don't see it being able to fill out forms without putting on a pitiful show of incompetence. That is not the appropriate time to bring out the creative genius.

Cooperate, you guys.

Supposedly long-term memory remains while short-term or newly learned information tends to evaporate. Sometimes that seems to be true as when my friend became a grandmother recently. She was worried that she wouldn't remember how to care for an infant but she said the knowledge came back instantly despite an almost thirty-year gap in practice. She had no trouble holding the baby the right way or changing a diaper. She burped her new grandchild like a pro and was a source of support for her daughter, as she had hoped to be.

But that isn't always the case. One woman I know who had, over the course of sixty years, propagated thousands of houseplants and now finds she can't remember their names. Surely her extended botanical history would qualify as long-term memory. It distresses her tremendously. What would it hurt for her brain to pitch in with stock from her archives?

I am having trouble remembering the tai chi moves I do every week. They are familiar as I do them in class but my retention goes home with my teacher. I admit to not practicing every day but I would think that after a couple of years the moves should have passed into kinetic if not cognitive memory.

Maybe it is as my friend says, that our brains are just overcrowded and something has to drop out. And maybe I'm being too hard on my brain, for at the same time I am forgetting, I find myself remembering. What I am remembering, however, is of a different quality. I may forget phone numbers but I remember concepts. Like how everyone is connected in some way and when we hurt someone else it usually ends up hurting us in return. Or how we have to be a good friend to have one. I remember that forgiving someone who hurt us frees up energy for loving ourselves. And I remember that we have a choice in how we experience life.

So if I have to deal with forgetting and remembering, I will do it on my own terms. It is my recipe for a good existence.

I choose to forget anything that hinders my appreciation of life.

I choose to remember all that makes being alive rich and wonderful.

A New Woman

I am rummaging around in my bathroom vanity looking for the loofah sponge that had somehow been shoved all the way to the back. I find it behind the towels, half-hidden under the extra bath mat. Next to a forgotten box of tampons.

I have cleaned this space since I stopped having my period. How can I have missed this?

I drag out the familiar box. How many boxes had I bought over how many years? Tampons accompanied me wherever I went. They were a staple of life. I would sooner have given up food than be without my tampons. Now I have no use for them.

I am about to toss the box into the trashcan beside the sink when I suddenly have to sit down. I am unprepared for the flood of emotions that washes over me.

Worry says, "Wait. You can't throw away the tampons, what if you need them?"

"Hah," laughs Relief. "You'll never need them again."

But, but, I stammer.

It all seemed so clear a second ago. No period, no need for tampons. Now I am curiously hesitant.

138

Maybe I shouldn't throw them out. After all, you can never be sure of anything.

"Don't be silly," pipes in Reason. "It's been over two years since you had your period. By all accounts, if you aren't bleeding for a year, you're done."

Right.

Once again I reach out to throw them away when Anxiety wonders, "Will you be giving up on your youth if you get rid of the major sign of a woman's vitality?"

"A tampon is only a tampon," says Reason. "Nothing else. Are you a woman or aren't you?

Anxiety has me concerned now. What if it's true? At this point in my life, the tampons are symbolic rather than useful but symbols are important. They help find meaning for the mysteries of life. By getting rid of the remaining symbols of my young womanhood, would I be moving on to be a crone or would it make me into a hag?

"Do you remember the first time you got your period?" creeps in Nostalgia with its seduction whine. "There wasn't anything as convenient as tampons then, only those big pads that never quite fit. Tampons made your life so much better."

"Pads, tampons, who cares?" says Comfort "You don't miss them one itsy, bitsy bit, be honest."

No, I don't miss them. I don't miss the cramps and the headaches that came with menstruation either. But do I miss that time of life? Would I want to be back there with its turmoil?

It isn't a realistic question because I can't go back even if I would choose to, but I am in the grip of Nostalgia and it doesn't give up easily.

"Wasn't it great when you could share your feelings with your friends who were going through the same thing?" Nostalgia continues. "They understood. They really knew what you were going through."

Yeah, friends are great, I concede. One friend and I have known each other since we were teens. We are old-time friends, we say, rather than old friends. We are very clear about our choice of words. What times we used to have.

"But you have friends now, too," says Compassion. "You probably have more close friends today than ever."

I do, I realize. I have friends, wonderful friends I have gathered over the course of more than forty years who comprise a support system that I value. We share our feelings freely. And with a lot of humor. It's hard to be serious when your face is dissolving in sweat. These friends not only understand what is going on at midlife, but address the issues with perspective and courage. And my old-time friendship is worth more to me than I could have imagined.

In fact, things are good at this age. I have more freedom to explore life with fewer encumbrances.

"Well," says Reason, "what are you going to do?"

All my emotions are waiting for my answer. In the stillness I know what needs to be done.

Intuition says quietly, "I will help you."

I take the tampons out of the box and one by one drop them into the waiting pail. Each one that falls bears a memory related to the girl I was, a tribute to the innocence I once had, or to the journey I have been traveling. Each receives a thank you for having accompanied me on my life's path. And each takes with it an ache or a sigh that might hold me back from progressing. When the box is empty, I crumple it and add it to the pile with my appreciation for it's facilitating this final release.

I have created my own ritual, a rite of passage to honor my maturing from fecund female to menopausal wise woman.

With the loofah in hand, I turn on my shower. I wash away any residue of regret or lingering wistfulness. My skin is invigorated, my spirit revived.

I am a new woman, ready for the future.

Epilogue
Where Am I Being?

It has taken years for this book to be written, years of physical changes and spiritual growth, of shifting perspectives and intermittent reality checks. I have often asked myself along the way, "Where am I going?" Sometimes I thought I knew but the path frequently turned out to be different from what I expected, leading me to unexplored places.

As I progress through midlife, I discover that I am not so much going as being. There is less pushing on my part and more allowing myself to be drawn. It is an interesting experience, quite in line with my spiritual philosophy. I see this drawing in large aspects and in everyday interactions.

It is happening in my family. My son and daughter are both now married. Their spouses bring additional energy, love, and fun into my life. They live further away than before, certainly not as close as I would like, but it seems that I am seeing them more. The dining room table keeps stretching to accommodate the expanding number of relatives. I have become an in-law and I find, contrary to stereotypes, that being an in-law is rather nice.

After years out of the teaching profession, I have been drawn into giving a course in children's writing at a local university. I didn't seek the job; it found me. The learning curve is steep, more for me than my students, as I have to break down what comes naturally to teach it to them. I am excited and nervous at the same time, but looking forward to a productive year and being a teacher again.

This summer I was adopted by a stray cat, a wonderful cat who didn't know I was allergic to animals. I tried to discourage the bond that seemed to be growing between us but I fell in love with this brown and black tabby with the black stripe down his back that made him look like a skunk. Loving my grandcat for short periods of time is not the same as living full time with a furry cat, no matter how sweet. I had to find a caring home for him before the harsh winter weather set in because I couldn't let him stay in my house. My ability to apply my lessons in letting go was tested as I tearfully handed him over to his new adoptive parents. Doing the right thing doesn't mean not being hurt.

Occasionally I turn into Swamp Woman, though not as frequently as I used to. She makes me laugh and shakes up the people in my life who forget she's around. I like being Swamp Woman. She reminds me of the creative possibilities within me.

So I am now asking myself a different question: "Where am I being today?"

Where am I experiencing myself? Am I being appreciative or unaware? Am I being swampy or on the roller coaster?

And where am I being tomorrow?

About the Author

Ferida Wolff started her writing career by freelancing as a feature writer for newspapers and magazines. She went on to write books for children, publishing with HarperCollins, Random House, Houghton Mifflin Company, Little Brown and Company, William Morrow, Scholastic Books and The Jewish Publication Society. Her essays have appeared in The New York Times, The Philadelphia Inquirer, Moment Magazine and Mature Years and she is a contributor to the Chicken Soup for the Soul and the Chocolate for the Woman's Soul series. Her first book for adults, *Listening Outside Listening Inside*, is a collection of inspirational stories about listening to our inner messages.